Clinical
Calculations
With Applications to General and Specialty Areas

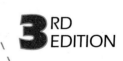

3RD
EDITION

Clinical Calculations

With Applications to General and Specialty Areas

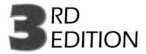

JOYCE L. KEE, RN, MS

Associate Professor Emerita
College of Nursing
University of Delaware
Newark, Delaware

SALLY M. MARSHALL, RN, MSN

Nursing Service
Department of Veterans Affairs
Regional Office and Medical Center
Wilmington, Delaware

3RD EDITION

W.B. SAUNDERS COMPANY
A Division of Harcourt Brace & Company
PHILADELPHIA LONDON TORONTO
MONTREAL SYDNEY TOKYO

W.B. SAUNDERS COMPANY
A Division of Harcourt Brace & Company

The Curtis Center
Independence Square West
Philadelphia, Pennsylvania 19106

Notice: The authors of this book have made every effort to ensure that the dosages of drugs are correct and in accordance with the standards accepted at the time of publication. The reader is advised to consult the instruction insert of each drug before administering to ascertain any change in drug dosage, method of administration, or contraindications. Because changes are continually occurring in the field and because of the fundamental importance of the specific circumstances and of the etiology of the patient's condition, it must be the responsibility of treating physicians, relying on their professional experience and their knowledge of the patient, to determine dosages and the best treatment for a patient.

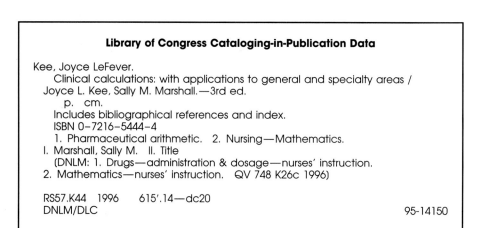

Library of Congress Cataloging-in-Publication Data

Kee, Joyce LeFever.
   Clinical calculations: with applications to general and specialty areas /
Joyce L. Kee, Sally M. Marshall.—3rd ed.
     p. cm.
   Includes bibliographical references and index.
   ISBN 0-7216-5444-4
    1. Pharmaceutical arithmetic. 2. Nursing—Mathematics.
I. Marshall, Sally M. II. Title
   (DNLM: 1. Drugs—administration & dosage—nurses' instruction.
2. Mathematics—nurses' instruction. QV 748 K26c 1996)

RS57.K44 1996   615'.14—dc20
DNLM/DLC   95-14150

CLINICAL CALCULATIONS: WITH APPLICATIONS TO
GENERAL AND SPECIALTY AREAS, THIRD EDITION   ISBN 0-7216-5444-4

Printed in the United States of America

Last digit is the print number: 9   8   7   6   5   4

To my mother
and
To my Children, Drew and Sarah
Sally Marshall

———————————

To my grandchildren
Christopher, Brenda, Jessica, and Kimberly
Joyce Kee

———————————

To our
nursing colleagues

Preface

This text arose from the need to bridge a learning gap between education and practice. We believe the this bridge is needed in order for the student to understand the wide range of clinical calculations used in nursing practice. This book provides a comprehensive application of calculations in nursing practice.

The last edition of *Clinical Calculations: With Applications to General and Specialty Areas* has been expanded in this third edition on topics in several areas to show the interrelationship between calculation and drug administration. Along with the chapter *Interpretation of Drug Labels, Drug Orders, Charting, ''5 Rights,'' and Abbreviations* which was added in the present edition, a new chapter related to drug administration, *Alternative Methods for Drug Administration,* is included.

The changes made in the third edition also include the following:

- In *Part One: Basic Math Review,* more practice problems are included on fractions, decimals, and percents; more questions are included in the Post-Math Test.

- An increased number of drug labels, illustrations, and tables are included throughout the text.

- The number of practice problems has increased by 25%.

- An increased number of practice problems using dimensional analysis as the calculation method are added in Chapters 5, 6, and 7. The basic formula and ratio and proportion are the major methods used throughout the text.

- The ''5 Rights'' with a checklist related to drug administration is included in the chapter, *Interpretation of Drug Labels, Drug Orders, Charting, ''5 Rights,'' and Abbreviations.*

- A new section on enteral feedings and medications with practice problems is included in Chapter 6, *Oral and Enteral Preparations with Clinical Applications.*

- The chapter on *Intravenous Preparations with Clinical Applications* was made. New illustrations are added including central venous line placements.

- Illustrations of intramuscular injection sites are added to the chapter *Injectable Preparations with Clinical Applications.*

- A new section on direct intravenous injection (IV push) with practice problems is included in the chapter *Injectable Preparations with Clinical Applications.*

- Additional cards, such as the *Check List of the "5 Rights," in Drug Administration,* are included at the end of the text. These cards can be detached from the book and carried in the nurse's uniform pocket.
- Testbank questions, in booklet form for instructors, are available.

Clinical Calculation is unique in that it has calculation problems for not only the general patient care areas, but also for the specialty units, pediatrics, critical care, pediatric critical care, labor and delivery, and community. The book is useful for nurses in all levels of nursing education who are learning for the first time how to calculate dosage problems and for beginning practitioners in specialty areas. It also can be used in nursing refresher courses, inservice programs, hospital units, home health care, and other places of nursing practice.

The book is divided into four parts. Part One is the basic math review, written concisely for nursing students to review Roman numerals, fractions, decimals, percentages, and ratio and proportion. A post-math review test follows. The math test can be taken first, and if the student has a score of 90% or higher, the basic review section can be omitted. Part Two covers metric, apothecary, and household systems used in drug calculations; conversion of units; reading drug labels, drug orders, and abbreviations; and methods of calculations. Part Three covers calculating drug and fluid dosages for oral, injectable, and intravenous administration. Clinical drug calculations used in specialty areas are found in Part Four. This part includes pediatrics, critical care for adults and children, labor and delivery, and community.

In the appendix, guidelines for administrations of medications (oral, injectable, and intravenous) are given. The index assists in locating content in the text.

Each chapter has a content list, objectives, introduction, and numerous practice problems. The practice problems are related to clinical drug problems that are currently used in clinical settings. Illustrations such as tablets, capsules, medicine cup, syringes, ampules, vials, intravenous bag and bottle, IV tubing, electronic IV devices, intramuscular injection sites, central venous sites, and many others are provided throughout the text.

Calculators may be used in solving dosage problems. Many institutions have calculators available. It is suggested that the nurse work the problem without a calculator and then check the answer with a calculator.

TO THE INSTRUCTOR: A suggestion on how this book may be used by the student: Assign Part One and Part Two which covers delivery of medication prior to the class. A testbank of questions is also available for the instructor's use.

Joyce L. Kee
Sally M. Marshall

Acknowledgments

We wish to extend our sincere appreciation to the individuals who have helped with this third edition: Adrienne Woods, RN, MSN, for her suggestions and use of her book, *Nurses' Drug Handbook,* by Sporatto and Woods; Janice Compton, RN, BSN; Melody Thorpe, RN, BSN; Rena Earnhart, RN, BSN; Mary Ellen Sweeny, RN, MSN; Carole McShane, RN, BSN; Janet Fanuele, RN, MSN; and Paul Schuele, HN, MICU; all from the Veterans Administration Medical Center, Wilmington, Delaware. Our thanks also goes to Ron Sweeny for his illustrations in this edition. We thank Don Passidomo, head librarian at the Veterans Administration Medical Center, for his assistance.

Our deepest appreciation goes to pharmaceutical companies for permission to use their drug labels. Pharmaceutical companies that extended their courtesy to this book include

Bristol-Myers Squibb Company
Squibb and Sons, Incorporated
Apothecon Laboratories
Princeton Pharmaceutical Products

Burroughs-Wellcome Company
(Reproduced with permission of Burroughs-Wellcome Company.)

Eli Lilly and Company

Lederle Laboratories *(Drug labels— Copyright, Lederle Laboratories, Division of American Cyanamid Company, all rights reserved. Reprinted with permission.)*

American Regent Laboratories, Incorporated
Luitpold Pharmaceuticals

Marion Merrell Dow, Incorporated

McNeilab, Incorporated
McNeil Consumer Products Company
McNeil Pharmaceutical

Merck and Company, Incorporated
Merck/DuPont Pharmaceuticals

Warner-Lambert Company
Parke-Davis Company
Warner Chilcott Laboratories

SmithKline Beecham Pharmaceuticals

Wyeth-Ayerst Laboratories *(Courtesy of Wyeth-Ayerst Laboratories.)*

We extend our sincere thanks to the various companies and publishers who gave us permission to use photographs, illustrations, and other materials in the text. These include

American Association of Critical Care Nursing

Appleton & Lange

Ciba-Geigy Pharmaceuticals

F. A. Davis

IMED Corporation

W. B. Saunders Company

Wyeth-Ayerst Laboratories

To the staff at W. B. Saunders, our sincere thanks for their suggestions and assistance.

We wish to extend our appreciation and love to our husbands, Edward D. Kee and Robert F. Marshall, for their support and suggestions.

Joyce L. Kee
Sally M. Marshall

Brief Contents

Contents

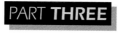

PART **FOUR**   **Calculations for Specialty Areas** ____ **189**

CHAPTER   9

CHAPTER   10

CHAPTER 11

CHAPTER 12

Basic Math Review

OBJECTIVES

- Convert Roman numerals to Arabic numbers.
- Multiply and divide fractions and decimals.
- Solve ratio and proportion problems.
- Change percentage to decimals, fractions, and ratio and proportion.
- Demonstrate an understanding of Roman numerals, fractions, decimals, ratio and proportion, and percentage by passing the math test.

The basic math review assists nurses in converting Roman and Arabic numerals, multiplying and dividing fractions and decimals, and solving ratio and proportion and percentage problems. Nurses need to master basic math skills to solve drug problems used in the administration of medication.

A math test, found on page 11, follows the basic math review. The test may be taken first, and if a score of 90% or greater is achieved, the math review, or Part I, can be omitted. If the test score is less than 90%, the nurse should do the basic math review section. Some nurses may choose to start with Part One and then take the test.

Answers to the Practice Problems are at the end of Part One, before the Post-Math Test.

NUMBER SYSTEMS

Two systems of numbers currently used are Arabic and Roman. Both systems are used in drug administration.

Arabic System

The Arabic system is expressed in numbers: 0, 1, 2, 3, 4, 5, 6, 7, 8, 9. These can be written as a whole number or with fractions and decimals. This system is commonly used today.

Roman System

Numbers used in the Roman system are designated by selected capital letters, i.e., I, V, X. Roman letters can be changed to Arabic numbers.

Conversion of Systems

ROMAN NUMBER	ARABIC NUMBER
I	1
V	5
X	10
L	50
C	100

The apothecary system of measurement uses Roman numerals when writing drug dosages. The Roman numerals are written in lower case letters, i.e., i, v, x, xii. The lower case letters can be topped by a horizontal line, i.e., ī, v̄, x̄, x̄īī

Roman numerals can appear together, such as xv and ix. To read multiple Roman numerals, addition and subtraction are used.

METHOD A

If the *first* Roman numeral is *greater* than the following numeral(s), then **ADD.**

$$\overline{VIII} = 5 + 3 = 8$$

$$\overline{XV} = 10 + 5 = 15$$

METHOD B   If the *first* Roman numeral is *less* than the following numeral(s), then **SUBTRACT.** Subtract the first numeral from the second (i.e., the smaller from the larger).

$$\overline{IV} = 5 - 1 = 4$$

$$\overline{IX} = 10 - 1 = 9$$

Some Roman numerals require both addition and subtraction to ascertain their value. Read from left to right.

$$\overline{XIX} = 10 + 9(10 - 1) = 19$$

$$\overline{XXXIV} = 30(10 + 10 + 10) + 4(5 - 1) = 34$$

I. Practice Problems: Roman Numerals

1. $\overline{XVI}$

_____

2. $\overline{XII}$

_____

3. $\overline{XXIV}$

_____

4. $\overline{XXXIX}$

_____

5. XLV

_____

6. XC

_____

FRACTIONS

Fractions are expressed as part(s) of a whole or part(s) of a unit. A fraction is composed of two basic numbers: a *numerator* (the top number) and a *denominator* (the bottom number). The denominator indicates the total number of parts

Fraction: $\underline{3}$ numerator (3 of 4 parts)

       4 denominator (4 of 4 parts, or 4 total parts)

The value of a fraction depends mainly on the denominator. When the denominator increases, for example, from $\frac{1}{10}$ to $\frac{1}{20}$, the value of the fraction decreases, because it takes more parts to make a whole.

EXAMPLE

Which fraction has the greater value: $\frac{1}{4}$ or $\frac{1}{6}$? The denominators are 4 and 6.

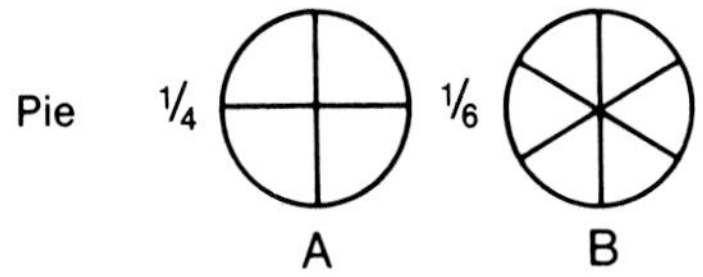

The larger value is $\frac{1}{4}$, because four parts make the whole, whereas for $\frac{1}{6}$, it takes six parts to make a whole. Therefore, $\frac{1}{6}$ has the smaller value.

Proper, Improper, and Mixed Fractions

In a *proper fraction* (simple fraction), the numerator is less than the denominator, i.e., $\frac{1}{2}$, $\frac{2}{3}$, $\frac{3}{4}$, $\frac{2}{6}$. When possible, the fraction should be reduced to its lowest term, i.e., $\frac{2}{6} = \frac{1}{3}$ (2 goes into 2 and 6).

In an *improper fraction,* the numerator is greater than the denominator, i.e., $\frac{4}{2}$, $\frac{8}{5}$, $\frac{14}{4}$. Reduce improper fractions to whole numbers or mixed numbers, i.e., $\frac{4}{2} = 2$ ($\frac{4}{2}$ means the same as $4 \div 2$); $\frac{8}{5} = 1\frac{3}{5}$ ($8 \div 5$, 5 goes into 8 one time with 3 left over, or $\frac{3}{5}$); and $\frac{14}{4} = 3\frac{2}{4} = 3\frac{1}{2}$ ($14 \div 4$, 4 goes into 14 three times with 2 left over, or $\frac{2}{4}$, which can then be reduced to $\frac{1}{2}$).

A *mixed number* is a whole number and a fraction, i.e., $1\frac{3}{5}$, $3\frac{1}{2}$. Mixed numbers can be changed to improper fractions by multiplying the denominator by the whole number, then adding the numerator, i.e., $1\frac{3}{5} = \frac{8}{5}$ ($5 \times 1 = 5, + 3 = 8$).

The apothecary system uses fractions to indicate drug dosages. Fractions may be added, subtracted, multiplied, or divided. Multiplying fractions and dividing fractions are the two common methods used in solving dosage problems.

Multiplying Fractions

To multiply fractions, multiply the numerators and then the denominators. Reduce the fraction, if possible, to lowest terms.

EXAMPLES

1. $\frac{1}{3} \times \frac{3}{5} = \frac{\overset{1}{\cancel{3}}}{\underset{5}{\cancel{15}}} = \frac{1}{5}$

The answer is $\frac{3}{15}$, which can be reduced to $\frac{1}{5}$. The number that goes into both 3 and 15 is 3. Therefore, 3 goes into 3 one time, and 3 goes into 15 five times.

2. $\frac{1}{3} \times 6 = \frac{6}{3} = 2$

A whole number can also be written as that number over one ($\frac{6}{1}$). Six is divided by 3 ($6 \div 3$); 3 goes into 6 two times.

Dividing Fractions

To divide fractions, invert the *second fraction,* or divisor, and then multiply.

EXAMPLES

1. $\frac{3}{4} \div \frac{3}{8}$ (divisor) $= \frac{\overset{1}{\cancel{3}}}{\underset{1}{\cancel{4}}} \times \frac{\overset{2}{\cancel{8}}}{\underset{1}{\cancel{3}}} = \frac{2}{1} = 2$

When dividing, invert the divisor 3/8 to 8/3 and multiply. To reduce the fraction to lowest terms, 3 goes into both 3s one time, and 4 goes into 4 and 8 one time and two times, respectively.

2. $\frac{1}{6} \div \frac{4}{18} = \frac{1}{\underset{1}{\cancel{6}}} \times \frac{\overset{3}{\cancel{18}}}{4} = \frac{3}{4}$

Six and 18 are reduced or canceled, to 1 and 3.

Decimal Fractions

Fractions can be changed to decimals. Divide the numerator by the denominator, i.e., $\frac{3}{4} = 4\overline{)3.00}$ = 0.75. Therefore, 3/4 is the same as 0.75.

1. a. Which has the greatest value: 1/50, 1/100, or 1/150? ____________

b. Which has the lowest value: 1/50, 1/100, or 1/150? ____________

2. Reduce improper fractions to whole or mixed numbers.

a. 12/4 = ____________

b. 20/5 = ____________

c. 22/3 = ____________

d. 32/6 = ____________

3. Multiply fractions.

a. 2/3 × 1/8 = ____________

b. 2 2/5 × 3 3/4 =
12/5 × 15/4 = ____________

c. 500/350 × 5 = ____________

d. 400,000/200,000 × 3 = ____________

4. Divide fractions.

a. 2/3 ÷ 6 = ____________

b. 1/4 ÷ 1/5 = ____________

c. 1/6 ÷ 1/8 = ____________

d. 1/150/1/100 = (1/150 ÷ 1/100) = ____________

e. 1/200 ÷ 1/300 = ____________

f. 9 3/5 ÷ 4 =
48/5 ÷ 4/1 = ____________

5. Change fraction to a decimal.

    a. ¼ =   **b.** ¹/₁₀ =   **c.** ²/₅ =

    _____   _____   _____

DECIMALS

Decimals consist of (1) whole numbers (numbers to the left of decimal point) and (2) decimal fractions (numbers to the right of decimal point). The following number, 2468.8642, is an example of the division of units for a whole number with a decimal fraction.

WHOLE NUMBERS					DECIMAL FRACTIONS			
2	4	6	8	•	8	6	4	2
Thousands	Hundreds	Tens	Units		Tenths	Hundredths	Thousandths	Ten Thousandths

Decimal fractions are written in tenths, hundredths, thousandths, and ten-thousandths. Frequently, decimal fractions are used in drug dosing. The metric system is referred to as the decimal system. After solving decimal problems, decimal fractions are rounded off to tenths. To round off to tenths, if the hundredth column is 5 or greater, the tenth is increased by 1, i.e., 0.67 is rounded up to 0.7 (tenths).

Decimal fractions are an integral part of the metric system. Tenths mean 0.1 or ¹/₁₀, hundredths mean 0.01 or ¹/₁₀₀, and thousandths mean 0.001 or ¹/₁₀₀₀. When a decimal is changed to a fraction, the denomination is based on the number of digits to the right of the decimal point (0.8 is ⁸/₁₀, 0.86 is ⁸⁶/₁₀₀)

EXAMPLES

1. 0.5 is ⁵/₁₀, or 5 tenths.

2. 0.55 is ⁵⁵/₁₀₀, or 55 hundredths.

3. 0.555 is ⁵⁵⁵/₁₀₀₀, or 555 thousandths.

Multiplying Decimals

To multiply decimal numbers, multiply the multiplicand by the multiplier. Count how many numbers (spaces) are to the right of the decimals in the problem. Mark off the number of decimal spaces in the answer (right to left) according to the number of decimal spaces in the problem. Round off in tenths.

EXAMPLE

$$
\begin{array}{r}
1.34 \quad \text{multiplicand} \\
2.3 \quad \text{multiplier} \\
\hline
402 \\
268\cancel{0} \\
\hline
3.082 \quad \text{or 3.1 (rounded off in tenths)}
\end{array}
$$

Answer: 3.1

Because 8 is greater than 5, the "tenth" number is increased by 1.

Dividing Decimals

To divide decimal numbers, the decimal point in the divisor is moved to the right to make a whole number. The decimal point in the dividend is also moved to the right according to the number of decimal spaces in the divisor.

EXAMPLE

Dividend ÷ Divisor

$$2.46 \div 1.2 \quad or \quad \frac{2.46}{1.2} =$$

$$
\begin{array}{r}
2.05 = 2.1 \\
(divisor) \ 1.2 \ \overline{)2.4 \ 60} \ (dividend) \\
\underline{2\ 4} \\
60 \\
\underline{60} \\
0
\end{array}
$$

III. Practice Problems: Decimals

1. Multiply decimals.
   a. 6.8 × 0.123 =   **b.** 52.4 × 9.345 =

_____   _____

2. Divide decimals.
   a. 69 ÷ 3.2 =   **c.** 100 ÷ 4.5 =

_____   _____

   b. 6.63 ÷ 0.23 =   **d.** 125 ÷ 0.75 =

_____   _____

3. Change decimals to fractions.
   a. 0.46 =   **b.** 0.05 =   **c.** 0.012 =

_____   _____   _____

4. Which has the greatest value: 0.46, 0.05, or 0.012? Which has the lowest value?

_____

RATIO AND PROPORTION

A _ratio_ is the relation between two numbers and is separated by a colon, i.e., 1 : 2 (1 is to 2). It is another way of expressing a fraction, i.e., 1 : 2 = ½.

Proportion is the relation between two ratios separated by a double colon (: :) or equal sign (=).

To solve a ratio and proportion problem, the middle numbers _(means)_ are multiplied and the end numbers _(extremes)_ are multiplied. To solve for the unknown, which is X, the X goes to the left side and is followed by an equal sign.

EXAMPLES

1. 1 : 2 : : 2 : X (1 is to 2, as 2 is to X)

    means

    extremes

      X = 4   (1 X is the same as X)

Answer: 4 (1 : 2 : : 2 : 4)

2. 4 : 8 = X : 12

   8 X = 48

    X = $^{48}/_8$ = 6

Answer: 6 (4 : 8 = 6 : 12)

3. A ratio and proportion problem may be set up as a fraction.

Ratio and Proportion	_Fraction_
2 : 3 : : 4 : X	$\frac{2}{3} = \frac{4}{X}$ (cross multiply)
2X = 12	2X = 12
X = $^{12}/_2$ = 6	X = 6

Answer: 6. Remember to cross-multiply when the problem is set up as a fraction.

IV. Practice Problems: Ratio and Proportion

Solve for X.

1. 2 : 10 : : 5 : X

_____

2. 0.9 : 100 = X : 1000

_____

3. Change ratio and proportion to fraction.
3 : 5 : : X : 10

_____

4. It is 500 miles from Washington, DC, to Boston, MA. Your car averages 22 miles per 1 gallon of gasoline. How many gallons of gasoline will be needed for the trip?

_____

PERCENTAGE

Percent (%) means 100. Two percent (2%) means 2 parts of 100, and 0.9% means 0.9 part (less than 1) of 100. A percent can be expressed as a fraction, a decimal, or a ratio.

EXAMPLE

Percent		Fraction	Decimal	Ratio
60%	=	$^{60}/_{100}$	0.60	60 : 100

Note: To change a percent to a decimal, move the decimal point two places to the left. In the example, the decimal point comes before the whole number 60.

V. Practice Problems: Percentage

Change percent to fraction, decimal, and ratio.

Percent	Fraction	Decimal	Ratio
1. 2%			
2. 0.33%			
3. 150%			
4. ½% (0.5%)			
5. 0.9%			

ANSWERS

I. Roman Numerals

1. 10 + 5 + 1 = 16
2. 10 + 2 = 12
3. 20(10 + 10) + 4(5 − 1) = 24
4. 30(10 + 10 + 10) + 9(10 − 1) = 39
5. 40(50 − 10) + 5 = 45
6. 100 − 10 = 90

II. Fractions

1. a. $\frac{1}{50}$ has the greatest value.   **b.** $\frac{1}{150}$ has the lowest value.

2. a. 3   **c.** $7\frac{1}{3}$

  b. 4   **d.** $5\frac{2}{6}$ or $5\frac{1}{3}$

3. a. $\frac{2}{24} = \frac{1}{12}$

  c. $\dfrac{\overset{10}{\cancel{500}}}{\underset{7}{\cancel{350}}} \times 5 = \dfrac{50}{7} = 7.1$

  b. $\frac{12}{5} \times \frac{15}{4} = \dfrac{180}{20} = 9$

  d. $\dfrac{\overset{2}{\cancel{400,000}}}{\underset{1}{\cancel{200,000}}} \times 3 = 6$

4. a. $\frac{2}{3} \div 6 = \frac{2}{3} \times \frac{1}{6}$

  $= \frac{2}{18} = \frac{1}{9}$

  d. $\frac{1}{150} \div \frac{1}{100} = \dfrac{1}{\underset{3}{\cancel{150}}} \times \dfrac{\overset{2}{\cancel{100}}}{1}$

  b. $\frac{1}{4} \div \frac{1}{5} =$

  $\frac{1}{4} \times \frac{5}{1} = \frac{5}{4} =$

  $1\frac{1}{4}$, or 1.25

  $= \frac{2}{3}$, or 0.666, or 0.67

  e. $\frac{1}{200} \div \frac{1}{300} = \frac{1}{200} \times \frac{300}{1} =$

  $\frac{300}{200} = 1\frac{1}{2}$, or 1.5

  c. $\dfrac{1}{6} \div \dfrac{1}{8} = \dfrac{1}{\underset{3}{\cancel{6}}} \times \dfrac{\overset{4}{\cancel{8}}}{1} = \dfrac{4}{3} = 1.33$

  f. $\frac{48}{5} \div \frac{4}{1} = \frac{48}{5} \times \frac{1}{4}$

  $= \dfrac{48}{20} = 2.4$

5. a. $\frac{1}{4} = 4\overline{)1.00}^{\,0.25}$ **b.** $\frac{1}{10} = 10\overline{)1.00}^{\,0.10}$ **c.** $\frac{2}{5} = 5\overline{)2.00}^{\,0.40}$

III. Decimals

1. a. 0.8364, or 0.8

  0.123
  6.8
  984
  738
  0.8364, or 0.8 (round off in tenths: 3 hundredths is less than 5)

  b. 489.6780, or 489.7 (7 hundredths is greater than 5)

2. a. 21.56, or 21.6 (6 hundredths is greater than 5, so the tenth is increased by one)

  b. 28.826, or 28.8 (2 hundredths is *not* 5 or greater than 5, so the tenth is not changed)

  c. $100 \div 4.5 = 4.5\overline{)100.0} = 22.2$, or 22

  d. $125 \div 0.75 = 0.75\overline{)125.00} = 166.6$, or 167

3. a. $\frac{46}{100}$ **b.** $\frac{5}{100}$ **c.** $\frac{12}{1000}$

4. 0.46 has the greatest value; 0.012 has the lowest value. Forty-six hundredths is greater than 5 hundredths or 12 thousandths.

IV. Ratio and Proportion

1. 2X = 50
  X = 25

2. 100X = 900
  X = 9

3. $\frac{3}{5} = \frac{X}{10} = 5X = 30$
  X = 6

4. 1 gal : 22 miles : : X gal : 500
  22X = 500
  X = 22.7 gal
  22.7 gallons of gasoline are needed

V. Percentage

	Percent	*Fraction*	*Decimal*	*Ratio*
1.	2	$^{2}/_{100}$	0.02	2 : 100
2.	0.33	$^{0.33}/_{100}$, or $^{33}/_{10,000}$	0.0033	0.33 : 100, or 33 : 10,000
3.	150	$^{150}/_{100}$	1.50	150 : 100
4.	0.5	$^{0.5}/_{100}$, or $^{5}/_{1000}$	0.005	0.5 : 100, or 5 : 1000
5.	0.9	$^{0.9}/_{100}$, or $^{9}/_{1000}$	0.009	0.9 : 100, or 9 : 1000

POST-MATH TEST

The math test is composed of five sections: Roman and Arabic numerals, fractions, decimals, ratios and proportions, and percentages. There are 60 questions. A passing score is 54 or more correct answers (90%). A nonpassing score is 7 or more incorrect answers.

Roman and Arabic Numerals

Convert Roman numerals to Arabic numerals.

1. $\overline{\text{vii}}$

2. $\overline{\text{xi}}$

3. $\overline{\text{xvi}}$

4. $\overline{\text{xiv}}$

5. xliii, or XLIII

Convert Arabic numerals to Roman numerals.

6. 4

7. 18

8. 29

9. 37

10. 62

Fractions

Which fraction has the larger value?

11. $^{1}/_{100}$ or $^{1}/_{150}$?

12. $^{1}/_{3}$ or $^{1}/_{2}$?

Reduce improper fractions to whole or mixed numbers.

13. $^{45}/_9 =$

14. $^{74}/_3 =$

Change mixed number to improper fraction.

15. $5^2/_3 =$

Change fractions to decimals.

16. $^2/_3 =$

17. $^1/_{12} =$

Multiply fractions.

18. $^7/_8 \times ^4/_6 =$

19. $2^3/_5 \times ^5/_8 =$

Divide fractions.

20. $^1/_2 \div ^1/_3 =$

22. $^1/_8 \div ^1/_{12} =$

21. $6^3/_4 \div 3 =$

23. $20^3/_4 \div ^1/_6 =$

Decimals

Round off decimal numbers to tenths.

24. $0.87 =$

26. $0.42 =$

25. $2.56 =$

Change decimals to fractions.

27. $0.68 =$

29. $0.012 =$

28. $0.9 =$

30. $0.33 =$

Multiply decimals.

31. $0.34 \times 0.6 =$

32. $2.123 \times 0.45 =$

_____

Divide decimals.

33. $3.24 \div 0.3 =$

_____

34. $69.4 \div 0.23 =$

_____

Ratio and Proportion

Change ratios to fractions.

35. $3 : 4 =$ **37.** $65 : 90 =$

_____   _____

36. $1 : 175 =$ **38.** $0.9 : 100 =$

_____   _____

Solve ratio and proportion problems.

39. $2 : 3 : : 8 : X$

_____

40. $0.5 : 20 : : X : 100$

_____

41. $3 : 100 = X : 1000$

_____

42. $5 : 25 = 10 : X$

_____

Change ratios and proportions to fractions and solve.

43. $1 : 2 : : 4 : X$

_____

44. $5 : 50 : : X : 300$

_____

45. $0.9 : 10 = X : 100$

_____

Percentage

Change percents to fractions.

46. $3\% =$ **47.** $27\% =$ **48.** $1.2\% =$ **49.** $5.75\% =$

Change percents to decimals.

50. 8% =   **52.** 0.9% =   **54.** 0.25% =
51. 15% =   **53.** 3.5% =   **55.** 0.45% =

Change percents to ratios.

56. 35% =   **58.** 4% =   **60.** 0.45% =
57. 12.5% =   **59.** 0.9% =

ANSWERS

Roman and Arabic Numerals

1. 7   **3.** 16   **5.** 43   **7.** $\overline{\text{XVIII}}$ **9.** $\overline{\text{XXXVII}}$
2. 11   **4.** 14   **6.** $\overline{\text{IV}}$ **8.** $\overline{\text{XXIX}}$ **10.** LXII

Fractions

11. $^1/_{100}$ **17.** 0.08   **20.** $\frac{1}{2} \times \frac{3}{1} =$ **22.** $\frac{1}{\cancel{8}} \times \frac{\cancel{12}^{\,3}}{1} =$
12. ½ $^3/_2 = 1\frac{1}{2}$ $\frac{2}{3}/2 = 1\frac{1}{2}$
13. 5   **18.** $\frac{28}{48}$ or $\frac{7}{12}$ $\frac{9}{}$
14. 24⅔
15. $^{17}/_3$ **19.** $\frac{13}{\cancel{5}^{\,1}} \times \frac{\cancel{5}}{8} =$ **21.** $\frac{\cancel{27}}{4} \times \frac{1}{\cancel{3}} =$ **23.** $\frac{83}{\cancel{4}_{\,2}} \times \frac{\cancel{6}^{\,3}}{1} =$
16. 0.66, or 0.7 $^{13}/_8 = 1^5/_8$ $\frac{9}{4} = 2\frac{1}{4}$ $^{249}/_2 = 124.5$

Decimals

24. 0.9   **27.** $^{68}/_{100}$ **30.** $\frac{33}{100}$ **33.** 10.8
25. 2.6   **28.** $^9/_{10}$ **31.** 0.204   **34.** 301.739, or
26. 0.4   **29.** $^{12}/_{1000}$ **32.** 0.95535, or   301.7
                                                    0.96, or 1.0

Ratio and Proportion

35. ¾   **41.** 30   **44.** $\frac{\cancel{5}^{\,1}}{\cancel{50}} = \frac{X}{300}$
36. $^1/_{175}$ **42.** 50 $10X = 300$
37. $^{65}/_{90}$ **43.** $\frac{1}{2} \times \frac{4}{x} =$ $X = 30$
38. $^9/_{1000}$ (cross multiply)   **45.** $^{0.9}/_{10} = ^X/_{100}$
39. 12 $X = 8$ $10X = 90$
40. 2.5 $X = 9$

Percentage

46. $^3/_{100}$ **51.** 0.15   **56.** 35 : 100
47. $^{27}/_{100}$ **52.** 0.009   **57.** 12.5 : 100, or
48. $^{12}/_{1000}$ **53.** 0.035   125 : 1000
49. $^{575}/_{10,000}$ **54.** 0.0025   **58.** 4 : 100
50. 0.08   **55.** 0.0045   **59.** 0.9 : 100, or 9 : 1000
                                                  60. 0.45 : 100, or
                                                      45 : 10,000

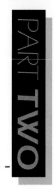

PART TWO

Systems, Conversion, and Methods of Drug Calculation

CHAPTER

Systems Used for Drug Administration

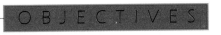

OBJECTIVES

- Recognize the system of measurement accepted world-wide and the system of measurement used in home settings.
- List the basic units and subunits of weight, volume, and length of the metric system.
- Explain the rules for changing grams to milligrams and milliliters to liters.
- Give abbreviations for the frequently used metric units and subunits.
- List the basic units in the apothecary system for weight and volume.
- Give the abbreviations for the apothecary and household units of measurement.
- List the basic units of measurement for volume in the household system.
- Convert units of measurement within the metric system, within the apothecary system, and within the household system.

The three systems used for measuring drugs and solutions are the metric, apothecary, and household. The metric system, developed in 1799 in France, is the chosen system for measurements in the majority of European countries. The metric system, also referred to as the decimal system, is based on units of 10. Since the enactment of the Metric Conversion Act of 1975, the United States has been moving toward the use of this system. The intention of the act is to adopt the International Metric System worldwide.

The apothecary system dates back to the Middle Ages and has been the system of weights and measurements used in England since the seventeenth century. This system is also referred to as the fractional system because anything less than one is expressed in fractions. In the United States, the apothecary system is rapidly being phased out and is being replaced with the metric system.

Standard household measurements are used primarily in home settings. With the trend toward home care, conversions to household measurements may gain importance.

METRIC SYSTEM

The metric system is a decimal system based on multiples of 10 and fractions of 10. There are three basic units of measurements. These basic units are:

Gram (g, gm, G, Gm) unit for weight

Liter (l, L) unit for volume or capacity

Meter (m, M) unit for linear measurement or length

Prefixes are used with the basic units to describe whether the units are larger or smaller than the basic unit. The prefixes indicate the size of the unit in multiples of 10. The prefixes for basic units are:

PREFIX FOR LARGER UNIT		PREFIX FOR SMALLER UNIT	
Kilo	1000 (one thousand)	Deci	0.1 (one-tenth)
Hecto	100 (one hundred)	Centi	0.01 (one-hundredth)
Deka	10 (ten)	Milli	0.001 (one-thousandth)
		Micro	0.000001 (one-millionth)
		Nano	0.000000001 (one-billionth)

Abbreviations of metric units that are frequently written in drug orders are listed in Table 1–1. Lowercase letters for abbreviations are usually used rather than capital letters.

The metric units of weight, volume, and length are given in Table 1–2. Meanings of the prefixes are stated next to the units of weight. Note that the larger units are 1000, 100, and 10 times the basic units (in bold type), and the smaller units differ by factors of 0.1, 0.01, 0.001, 0.000001, and 0.000000001. The size of a basic unit can be changed by multiplying or dividing by 10. Micrograms and nanograms are the exceptions: one (1) milligram = 1000 micrograms, and one (1) microgram = 1000 nanograms. Micrograms and nanograms are changed by 1000 instead of by 10.

TABLE 1–1
Metric Units and Abbreviations

	NAMES	ABBREVIATIONS
Weight	Kilogram	kg, Kg
	Gram	g, gm, G, Gm
	Milligram	mg, mgm
	Microgram	mcg, μg
	Nanogram	ng
Volume	Kiloliter	kl, kL
	Liter	l, L
	Deciliter	dl, dL
	Milliliter	ml, mL
Length	Kilometer	km, Km
	Meter	m, M
	Centimeter	cm
	Millimeter	mm

Conversion Within the Metric System

Drug administration often requires conversion within the metric system to prepare the correct dosage. Two basic methods are given for changing larger to smaller units and smaller to larger units.

METHOD A

To change from a **larger** unit to a **smaller** unit, *multiply by 10 for each unit decreased or* move the decimal point *one space to the right* for each unit changed.

TABLE 1–2
Units of Measurement in the Metric System with Their Prefixes

WEIGHT PER GRAM	MEANING
1 kilogram (kg) = 1000 grams	One thousand
1 hectogram (hg) = 100 grams	One hundred
1 dekagram (dag) = 10 grams	Ten
1 gram (g) = 1 gram	One
1 decigram (dg) = 0.1 gram ($^{1}/_{10}$)	One-tenth
1 centigram (cg) = 0.01 gram ($^{1}/_{100}$)	One-hundredth
1 milligram (mg) = 0.001 gram ($^{1}/_{1000}$)	One-thousandth
1 microgram (mcg) = 0.000001 gram ($^{1}/_{1,000,000}$)	One-millionth
1 nanogram (ng) = 0.000000001 gram ($^{1}/_{1,000,000,000}$)	One-billionth

VOLUME PER LITER	LENGTH PER METER
1 kiloliter (kL) = 1000 liters	1 kilometer (km) = 1000 meters
1 hectoliter (hL) = 100 liters	1 hectometer (hm) = 100 meters
1 dekaliter (daL) = 10 liters	1 dekameter (dam) = 10 meters
1 liter (l, L) = 1 liter	**1 meter (m) = 1 meter**
1 deciliter (dL) = 0.1 liter	1 decimeter (dm) = 0.1 meter
1 centiliter (cL) = 0.01 liter	1 centimeter (cm) = 0.01 meter
1 milliliter (mL) = 0.001 liter	1 millimeter (mm) = 0.001 meter

When changing three units from larger to smaller, such as from gram to milligram (a change of three units), multiply by 10 three times (or by 1000) or move the decimal point three spaces to the right.

Change 1 gram (g) to milligrams (mg).

    a. $1 \times \underline{10} \quad \times \underline{10} \quad \times \underline{10} \quad = 1000$ mg

    b. 1 g $\times$ 1000 = 1000 mg

             or

    c. 1 g = 1.000 mg (1000 mg)

When changing two units, such as kilogram to dekagram (a change of two units from larger to smaller), multiply by 10 twice (or by 100) or move the decimal point two spaces to the right.

Change 2 kilograms (kg) to dekagrams (dag).

    a. $2 \times \underline{10} \quad \times \underline{10} \quad = 200$ dag

    b. 2 kg $\times$ 100 = 200 dag

             or

    c. 2 kg = 2.00 dag (200 dag)

When changing one unit, such as liter to deciliter (a change of one unit from larger to smaller), multiply by 10 or move the decimal point one space to the right.

Change 3 liters (L) to deciliters (dL).

    a. 3 $\times$ 10 = 30 dL

    b. 3 L $\times$ 10 = 30 dL

             or

    c. 3 L = 3.0 dL (30 dL)

A micro unit is one-thousandth of a milli unit, and a nano unit is one-thousandth of a micro unit. Unit change of micro and nano to its nearest unit is done by multiplying by 1000 instead of by 10. When changing milli units to micro units, multiply by 1000 or move the decimal point three spaces to the right. The same is true when changing micro units to nano units.

EXAMPLES

PROBLEM 1: Change 2 grams (g) to milligrams (mg).

$$2 \text{ g} \times 1000 = 2000 \text{ mg}$$

or

$$2 \text{ g} = 2.000 \text{ mg} (2000 \text{ mg})$$

PROBLEM 2: Change 10 milligrams (mg) to micrograms (mcg).

$$10 \text{ mg} \times 1000 = 10,000 \text{ mcg} (\mu g)$$

or

$$10 \text{ mg} = 10.000 \text{ mcg} (10,000 \text{ mcg})$$

PROBLEM 3: Change 4 liters (L) to milliliters (mL).

$$4\ L \times 1000 = 4000\ mL$$

or

$$4\ L = 4.\underset{\curvearrowright}{000}\ mL\ (4000\ mL)$$

PROBLEM 4: Change 2 kilometers (km) to hectometers (hm).

$$2\ km \times 10 = 20\ hm$$

or

$$2\ km = 2.\underset{\curvearrowleft}{0}\ hm\ (20\ hm)$$

METHOD B

To change from a **smaller** unit to a **larger** unit, *divide by 10 for each unit increased or* move the decimal point *one space to the left* for each unit changed.

When changing three units from smaller to larger, divide by 1000 or move the decimal point three spaces to the left.

Change 1500 milliliters (mL) to liters (L).

a. $1500\ mL \div 1000 = 1.5\ L$

or

b. $1500\ mL = 1\ \underset{\curvearrowleft}{500}.\ L\ (1.5\ L)$

When changing two units from smaller to larger, divide by 100 or move the decimal point two spaces to the left.

Change 400 centimeters (cm) to meters (m).

a. $400\ cm \div 100 = 4\ m$

or

b. $400\ cm = 4\ \underset{\curvearrowleft}{00}.\ m\ (4\ m)$

When changing one unit from smaller to larger, divide by 10 or move the decimal point one space to the left.

Change 150 decigrams (dg) to grams (g).

a. $150\ dg \div 10 = 15\ g$

or

b. $150\ dg = 15\ \underset{\curvearrowleft}{0}.\ g\ (15\ g)$

EXAMPLES

PROBLEM 1: Change 8 grams to kilograms (kg).

$$8\ g \div 1000 = 0.008\ kg$$

or

$$8\ g = \underset{\curvearrowleft}{008}.\ kg\ (0.008\ kg)$$

PROBLEM 2: Change 1500 milligrams (mg) to decigrams (dg).

1500 mg ÷ 100 = 15 dg

or

1500 mg = 15 00. dg (15 dg)

PROBLEM 3: Change 750 micrograms (mcg) to milligrams (mg).

750 mcg ÷ 1000 = 0.75 mg

or

750 mcg = 750. mg (0.75 mg)

PROBLEM 4: Change 2400 milliliters (mL) to liters (L).

2400 ml ÷ 1000 = 2.4 L

or

2400 ml = 2 400. L (2.4 L)

I. Practice Problems: Metric Conversions

1. Conversion from larger units to smaller units: *multiply* by 10 for each unit changed (multiply by 10, 100, 1000) or move the decimal point one space to the *right* for each unit changed (move one, two, or three spaces), Method A. Answers are found on page 28.

   a. 7.5 grams to milligrams

   _____

   b. 10 milligrams to micrograms

   _____

   c. 35 kilograms to grams

   _____

   d. 2.5 liters to milliliters

   _____

   e. 1.25 liters to milliliters

   _____

   f. 20 centiliters to milliliters

   _____

   g. 18 decigrams to milligrams

   _____

   h. 0.5 kilograms to grams

   _____

2. Conversion from smaller units to larger units: *divide* by 10 for each unit changed (divide by 10, 100, 1000) or move the decimal point one space to the *left* for each unit changed (move one, two, or three spaces), Method B. Answers are found on page 28.

a. 500 milligrams to grams

_____

b. 7500 micrograms to milligrams

_____

c. 250 grams to kilograms

_____

d. 4000 milliliters to liters

_____

e. 325 milligrams to grams

_____

f. 100 milliliters to deciliters

_____

g. 2800 milliliters to liters

_____

h. 75 millimeters to centimeters

_____

APOTHECARY SYSTEM

The basic unit of weight in the apothecary system is the grain (gr), and the basic unit of fluid volume is the minim (℥); these are the smaller units in the apothecary system. Larger units of measurements for weight and fluid volume are the dram (dr or ℨ) and the ounce (oz or ℥). In the apothecary system, Roman numerals are written in lower case letters, e.g., gr x, to express numbers.

Table 1–3 gives the equivalents of units of dry weight (grain, dram, ounce) and units of liquid volume (minim, fluid dram, fluid ounce). The apothecary system uses fluid ounces and fluid drams to differentiate between liquid volume and dry weight. In clinical practice, units of liquid volume are commonly seen as dram and ounce. Often, the term fluid, which is the correct labeling of liquid volume, is dropped. However, the proper names for units of dry weight and units of liquid volume are used in this text.

The apothecary system is being phased out, and in the near future, all measurements will be in the metric system. Because there are physicians who still write medication orders using apothecary units, and probably will be for the next several decades, nurses need to know and to be able to interpret the apothecary system.

Conversion Within the Apothecary System

It is often necessary to change units within the apothecary system. The method applied when changing larger units to smaller units is:

TABLE 1-3
Abbreviations and Units of Measurement in the Apothecary System
----

ABBREVIATIONS

Weight		Liquid Volume	
grain	gr	quart	qt
ounce	oz, ʒ	pint	pt
dram	dr, ʒ	fluid ounce	fl oz, fl ʒ
		fluid dram	fl dr, fl ʒ
		minim	♏

BASIC EQUIVALENT UNITS

Weight			Liquid Volume*		
Larger units		*Smaller units*	*Larger units*		*Smaller units*
1 ounce	=	480 grains	1 quart	=	2 pints
1 ounce	=	8 drams	1 pint	=	16 fluid ounces
†1 dram	=	60 grains	1 fluid ounce	=	8 fluid drams
			1 fluid dram	=	60 minims
			†1 minim	=	1 drop (gt)

* Liquid volume of basic units is frequently used.
† Drams and minims are rarely used for drug administration; however, know their symbols.
Note: Constant values are the numbers of the smaller equivalent units.

METHOD C To change a **larger** unit to a **smaller** unit, *multiply* the constant value found in Table 1–3 by the number of the larger unit.

Note The constant values are the basic equivalent numbers of the smaller units given in Table 1–3. You might want to memorize these equivalents or refer to the table as needed.

EXAMPLES

PROBLEM 1: 2 drams (dr) = _____ grains (gr).

$$1 \text{ dr} = 60 \text{ gr (60 is the constant value, dry weight)}$$

$$2 \times 60 = 120 \text{ gr}$$

PROBLEM 2: 3 pints (pt) = _____ fluid ounces (fl oz or fl ʒ).

$$1 \text{ pt} = 16 \text{ fl oz (16 is the constant value)}$$

$$3 \times 16 = 48 \text{ fl oz, fl ʒ}$$

PROBLEM 3: 3 fluid ounces (fl ʒ) = _____ fluid drams (fl ʒ).

$$1 \text{ fl oz} = 8 \text{ fl dr (8 is the constant value)}$$

$$3 \times 8 = 24 \text{ fl dr, fl ʒ}$$

PROBLEM 4: 4 fluid drams (fl dr, fl ʒ) = _____ minims (♏).

1 fl dr = 60 minims (60 is the constant value)

4 × 60 = 240 ♏

The method applied when changing smaller units to larger units is:

METHOD D

To change a **smaller** unit to a **larger** unit, *divide* the constant value found in Table 1–3 by the number of the smaller unit.

EXAMPLES

PROBLEM 1: 30 grains (gr) = _____ dram (dr or ʒ).

1 dr = 60 gr (60 is the constant value)

30 ÷ 60 = ½ dr

PROBLEM 2: 80 fluid ounces (fl oz, fl ʒ) = _____ pints (pt).

1 pt = 16 fl oz (16 is the constant value)

80 ÷ 16 = 5 pts

PROBLEM 3: 2 fluid drams (fl dr, fl ʒ) = _____ fluid ounces (fl oz, fl ʒ).

1 fl oz = 8 fl dr (8 is the constant value)

2 ÷ 8 = ¼ fl oz

PROBLEM 4: 180 minims (♏) = _____ fluid drams (fl dr, fl ʒ).

1 fl dr = 60 minims (60 is the constant value)

180 ÷ 60 = 3 fl dr

II. Practice Problems: Apothecary System

Answers are found on page 28.

1. Give the abbreviations for:

   a. grain = _____
   b. dram = _____
   c. fluid dram = _____
   d. minim = _____
   e. drop = _____
   f. fluid ounce = _____
   g. pint = _____
   h. quart = _____

2. Give the equivalent using Method C, changing larger units to smaller units.

a. ℥ v = _____ gr

b. fl ℥ (fl oz) v = _____ fl ʒ (fl dr)

c. qt iii = _____ pt

d. pt ii = _____ fl ℥ (fl oz)

e. fl ʒ (fl dr) iiss = _____ ♏

3. Give the equivalent using Method D, changing smaller units to larger units.

a. gr 240 = _____ dr or ʒ

b. ʒ xvi = _____ oz or ℥

c. fl ʒ (fl dr) xxiv = _____ fl ℥ (fl oz)

d. ♏ xxx = _____ fl ʒ (fl dr)

e. ♏ xv = _____ gtt

HOUSEHOLD SYSTEM

The use of household measurements is on the increase because more patients/clients are being cared for in the home. The household system of measurement is not as accurate as the metric system because of a lack of standardization of spoons, cups, and glasses. A teaspoon (t) is considered 5 mL, although it could be anywhere from 4 to 6 mL. Three household teaspoons are equal to one tablespoon (T). A drop size can vary with the size of the lumen of the dropper. Basically, a drop and a minim are considered equal. Again, household measurements must be considered approximate measurements. Some of the household units are the same as the apothecary units, because there is a blend of these two systems.

The community health nurse may use and teach the household units of measurements to patients/clients.

Table 1–4 gives the commonly used units of measurement in the household system. You might want to memorize the equivalents in Table 1–4 or refer to the table as needed.

Conversion Within the Household System

For changing larger units to smaller units and smaller units to larger units within the household system, the same methods that applied to the apothecary system can be used. With household measurements, a fluid ounce is usually indicated as ounce.

TABLE 1–4
Units of Measurement in the Household System

1 drop (gt)	= 1 minim (♏)
1 teaspoon (t)	= 60 drops (gtt), 5 mL
1 tablespoon (T)	= 3 teaspoons (t)
1 ounce (oz)	= 2 tablespoons (T)
1 coffee cup (c)	= 6 ounces (oz)
1 medium size glass	= 8 ounces (oz)
1 measuring cup	= 8 ounces (oz)

Note: Constant values are the numbers of the smaller equivalent units.

METHOD E

To change a **larger** unit to a **smaller** unit, *multiply* the constant value found in Table 1–4 by the number of the larger unit.

Note The constant values are the basic equivalent numbers of the smaller units in Table 1–4.

EXAMPLES

PROBLEM 1: 2 medium size glasses = _____ ounces (oz).

    1 medium glass = 8 fl oz (8 is the constant value)

    $2 \times 8 = 16$ oz

PROBLEM 2: 3 tablespoons (T) = _____ teaspoons (t).

    1 T = 3 t (3 is the constant value)

    $3 \times 3 = 9$ t

PROBLEM 3: 5 ounces (oz or ℨ) = _____ tablespoons (T).

    1 oz = 2 T (2 is the constant value)

    $5 \times 2 = 10$ T

PROBLEM 4: 2 teaspoons (t) = _____ drops (gtt).

    1 t = 60 gtt (60 is the constant value)

    $2 \times 60 = 120$ gtt

METHOD F

To change a **smaller** unit to a **larger** unit, *divide* the constant value found in Table 1–4 into the number of the smaller unit.

EXAMPLES

PROBLEM 1: 120 drops (gtt) = _____ teaspoons (t).

    1 t = 60 gtt (60 is the constant value)

    $120 \div 60 = 2$ t

PROBLEM 2: 6 teaspoons (t) = _____ tablespoons (T).

    1 T = 3 t (3 is the constant value)

    $6 \div 3 = 2$ T

PROBLEM 3: 18 ounces (oz) = _____ cups (c).

    1 c = 6 oz (6 is the constant value)

    $18 \div 6 = 3$ c

PROBLEM 4: 4 tablespoons (T) = _____ ounces (oz).

1 oz = 2 T (2 is the constant value)

4 ÷ 2 = 2 oz

III. Practice Problems: Household System

1. Give the equivalents using Method E, changing larger units to smaller units.

a. 2 glasses = _____ oz

b. 3 ounces = _____ T

c. 4 tablespoons = _____ t

d. 1½ cups = _____ oz

e. ½ teaspoon = _____ gtt

2. Give the equivalents using Method F, changing smaller units to larger units.

a. 9 teaspoons = _____ T

b. 6 tablespoons = _____ oz

c. 90 drops = _____ t

d. 12 ounces = _____ c

e. 24 ounces = _____ medium size glasses

ANSWERS

I. Metric Conversions

1. a. 7.5 g to mg
7.5 g × 1000 = 7500 mg
or
7.500 mg (7500 mg)

b. 10,000 mcg
c. 35,000 g
d. 2500 mL
e. 1250 mL
f. 200 mL
g. 1800 mg
h. 500 g

2. a. 500 mg to g
500 ÷ 1000 = 0.5 g
or
500 mg = 500. g (0.5 g)

b. 7.5 mg
c. 0.25 kg
d. 4 L
e. 0.325 g
f. 1 dL
g. 2.8 L
h. 7.5 cm

II. Apothecary System

	Abbreviations	*Equivalents*	*Equivalents*
1. a.	grain = gr	**2. a.** ℥ v = _____ gr	**3. a.** gr 240 = _____ dr
b.	dram = dr or ʒ	5 × 60 = 300 gr	240 ÷ 60 = 4 dr or ʒ
c.	fluid dram = fl ʒ, fl dr	**b.** 40 fl ʒ, fl dr	**b.** 2 oz or ℥
d.	minim = ♏	**c.** 6 pt	**c.** 3 fl ℥, fl oz
e.	drop = gt	**d.** 32 fl ℥, fl oz	**d.** ½ fl ʒ, fl dr
f.	fluid ounce = fl ℥, fl oz	**e.** 150 ♏	**e.** 15 gtt
g.	pint = pt		
h.	quart = qt		

III. Household System

1. a. 2 glasses = _____ oz
   $2 \times 8 = 16$ oz
   b. 6 T
   c. 12 t
   d. 9 oz
   e. 30 gtt

2. a. 9 teaspoons = _____ T
   $9 \div 3 = 3$ T
   b. 3 oz
   c. 1½ t
   d. 2 c
   e. 3 glasses

SUMMARY PRACTICE PROBLEMS

1. Metric system
   a. 30 mg = _____ mcg (µg)
   b. 3 g = _____ mg
   c. 6 L = _____ mL
   d. 1.5 kg = _____ g
   e. 10,000 mcg = _____ mg
   f. 500 mg = _____ g
   g. 2500 mL = _____ L
   h. 125 g = _____ kg
   i. 120 mm = _____ cm
   j. 5 m = _____ cm

2. Apothecary system
   a. 90 gr = _____ dr
   b. fl ʒ (fl dr) iv = _____ fl ʒ (fl oz)
   c. fl ʒ (fl oz) iss = _____ fl ʒ (fl dr)
   d. ♏ xxx = _____ fl ʒ (fl dr)
   e. 8 pt = _____ qt
   f. fl ʒ (fl dr) ii = _____ ♏

3. Household system
   a. 12 t = _____ T
   b. 5 glasses = _____ oz
   c. 3 T = _____ t
   d. 2 c = _____ oz
   e. 30 oz = _____ c
   f. 4 oz = _____ T
   g. 12 gtt = _____ ♏

ANSWERS: SUMMARY PRACTICE PROBLEMS

1. a. 30,000 mcg
   b. 3000 mg
   c. 6000 mL
   d. 1500 g
   e. 10 mg

   f. 0.5 g
   g. 2.5 L
   h. 0.125 kg
   i. 12 cm
   j. 500 cm

2. a. 1.5 ℨ
  b. ½ or s̄s̄ fl ℥ (fl oz)
  c. 20 fl ℨ (fl dr)
  d. ½ or s̄s̄ fl ℨ (fl dr)
  e. 4 qt
  f. 120 ♏︎

3. a. 4 T
  b. 40 oz
  c. 9 t
  d. 12 oz
  e. 5 c
  f. 8 T
  g. 12 ♏︎

Conversion Within the Metric, Apothecary, and Household Systems

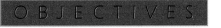

OBJECTIVES

- State rules for converting drug dosage by weight between the apothecary and metric systems.
- Convert grams/milligrams to grains and grains to grams/milligrams.
- Convert drug dosage by weight from one system to another system using the ratio method.
- State rules for converting drug dosage by volume among the metric, apothecary, and household systems.
- Convert liters/milliliters to ounces/pints and milliliters to drams, tablespoons, and teaspoons.

Drug doses are usually ordered in metric units (grams, milligrams, liters, and milliliters). Although the apothecary system is being phased out, there are some physicians who still order drug doses by apothecary units. To calculate a drug dose, the same unit of measurement must be used. Therefore, the nurse must know the metric and apothecary equivalents either by memorizing a conversion table or by using methods for converting from one system to the other. After the conversion is made, the dosage problem can be solved. Some authorities state it is easier to *convert to the unit used on the container (bottle)*. If the physician ordered phenobarbital gr ½ and the bottle is labeled 30 mg, then the conversion would be from grains to milligrams.

Metric and apothecary equivalents are approximations, e.g., 1 gram equals 15.432 grains. When values are unequal, they should be rounded off to the nearest whole number (1 gram = 15 grains).

Dosage conversion tables are available in many institutions; however, when you need a conversion table, one might not be available. Nurses should either memorize metric and apothecary equivalents or be able to convert from one system to the other by using calculation methods.

UNITS, MILLIEQUIVALENTS, AND PERCENTS

Units, milliequivalents, and percents are measurements used to indicate the strength or potency of certain drugs. When all drugs are developed, their strength is based on either chemical assay or biological assay. Chemical assay denotes strength by weight, e.g., milligrams or grains. Biological assays are used for drugs in which the chemical composition is difficult to determine. Biological assays assess potency by the effect one unit of the drug can have on a laboratory animal. Units mainly measure the potency of hormones, vitamins, anticoagulants, and some antibiotics. Drugs that were once standardized by units and later synthesized to their chemical composition may still retain units as an indication of potency, e.g., insulin.

Milliequivalents measure the strength of an ion concentration. Ions are given primarily for electrolyte replacement. They are measured in milliequivalents, mEq, which is $\frac{1}{1000}$ of the equivalent weight of an ion. Potassium chloride, KCl, is a common electrolyte replacement and is ordered in mEq.

Percents are the concentrations of weight dissolved in a volume and are always expressed as units of mass per units of volume. Common concentrations are g/mL, g/L or mg/mL. These concentrations, expressed as percentages, are based on the definition of a 1% solution as 1 g of a drug in 100 mL of solution. Dextrose 50% in a 50-mL pre-filled syringe is a concentration of 50 g of dextrose in 100 mL of water. Calcium gluconate 10% in a 30-mL bottle is a concentration of 10 g of calcium gluconate in 100 mL of solution. Proportions can also express concentrations. A solution that is 1 : 100 has the same concentration as a 1% solution. Epinephrine 1 : 1000 means that 1 g of epinephrine was dissolved in a 1000-mL solution.

Units, milliequivalents, and percents cannot be directly converted into the metric, apothecary, or household systems.

METRIC, APOTHECARY, AND HOUSEHOLD EQUIVALENTS

Knowing how to convert drug doses among the systems of measurement is essential in the clinical setting. In discharge teaching for individuals receiving liquid medication, converting metric to household measurement may be important.

Table 2–1 gives the metric and apothecary equivalents by weight and the metric, apothecary, and household equivalents by volume.

Remember, conversion from one system to another is an approximate equivalent. Either memorize Table 2–1 or use the methods that follow in the text for system conversion.

Conversion in Metric and Apothecary Systems by WEIGHT

GRAMS AND GRAINS 1 g = 15 gr

a. To convert grams to grains, *multiply* the number of grams by 15, the constant value.
b. To convert grains to grams, *divide* the number of grains by 15, the constant value.

TABLE 2–1
Approximate Metric, Apothecary, and Household Equivalents

	METRIC SYSTEM	**APOTHECARY SYSTEM**	**HOUSEHOLD SYSTEM**
Weight	30 g	1 oz	
	15 g	4 dr	
	*1 g; 1000 mg	15 (16) gr	
	0.5 g; 500 mg	7½ gr	
	0.3 g; 300 mg	5 gr	
	0.1 g; 100 mg	1½ gr	
	*0.06 g; 60 (65) mg	1 gr	
	0.03 g; 30 (32) mg	½ gr	
	0.01 g; 10 mg	⅙ gr	
	0.6 mg	$\frac{1}{100}$ gr	
	0.4 mg	$\frac{1}{150}$ gr	
	0.3 mg	$\frac{1}{200}$ gr	
Volume	1 L; 1000 mL (cc)	1 qt; 32 fl oz (fl ℥)	1 qt
	0.5 L; 500 mL	1 pt; 16 fl oz	1 pt
	0.24 L; 240 mL	8 oz	1 glass
	0.18 L; 180 mL	6 oz	1 c
	*30 mL	1 oz or 8 dr (fl ℥)	2 T or 6 t
	15 mL	½ oz or 4 dr	1 T
	4–5 mL		1 t
	4 mL	1 dr or 60 minims (♏)	1 t
	1 mL	15 (16) ♏	15–16 gtt
Other	1 kg; 1000 g	2.2 lb	

* Equivalents commonly used for computing conversion problems by ratio.
Note: ½ may be written as s̄s̄.

EXAMPLES

PROBLEM 1: Change 2 grams to grains.

$$2 \times 15 = 30 \text{ gr (grains)}$$

PROBLEM 2: Change 60 grains to grams.

$$60 \div 15 = 4 \text{ g (grams)}$$

GRAINS AND MILLIGRAMS   1 gr = 60 mg

    a. To convert grains to milligrams, *multiply* the number of grains by 60, the constant value.
    b. To convert milligrams to grains, *divide* the number of milligrams by 60, the constant value.

EXAMPLES

PROBLEM 1: Change 3 grains to milligrams.

$$3 \times 60 = 180 \text{ mg (milligrams)}$$

PROBLEM 2: Change 300 milligrams to grains.

Note 325 milligrams may be ordered instead of 300. Round off to the whole number. One grain is equivalent to 60, 64, or 65 milligrams. In this situation, you may want to divide by 65 instead of rounding off to the whole number.

$$300 \div 60 = 5 \text{ gr (grains)}$$

or

$$325 \div 65 = 5 \text{ gr}$$

or

$$325 \div 60 = 5.43 \text{ gr, or 5 gr (0.43 is less than 0.5)}$$

    If it is difficult for you to recall these methods, then use the ratio and proportion method to convert from one system to another.
    You must MEMORIZE:

1 gram = 1000 milligrams
1 gram = 15 grains
1 grain = 60 milligrams

Ratio and Proportion Multiply the means (numbers that are closest to each other) by the extremes (numbers that are farthest from each other). You are solving for X, so it goes first.

EXAMPLES

PROBLEM 1: Convert 2.5 grams to grains.

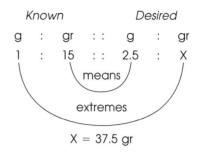

X = 37.5 gr

PROBLEM 2: Convert 10 grains to milligrams.

Known		Desired	
gr : mg	::	gr : mg	
1 : 60 (65)	::	10 : X	

X = 600 mg or 650 mg

Note Because conversion gives approximate values, the answer could be 600 mg or 650 mg. If the problem uses 1 gr = 60 mg, the answer is 600 mg. However, the bottle may be labeled 10 gr = 650 mg. Both 600 mg and 650 mg are correct.

I. Practice Problems: Conversion by Weight

Answers are found on page 38.

Grams and Grains

1. 10 g = _____ gr   **4.** 0.03 g = _____ gr
2. 0.5 g = _____ gr   **5.** 3 gr = _____ g
3. 0.1 g = _____ gr   **6.** 1½ gr = _____ g

Grains and Milligrams

1. 4 gr = _____ mg   **5.** 150 mg = _____ gr
2. 1½ gr = _____ mg   **6.** 30 mg = _____ gr
3. 7½ gr = _____ mg   **7.** 15 mg = _____ gr
4. ½ gr = _____ mg   **8.** 0.6 mg = _____ gr

Ratio and Proportion: Grams, Milligrams, and Grains

1. 2.5 g = _____ mg   **4.** 500 mg = _____ g
2. 0.5 g = _____ gr   **5.** 1 gr = _____ g
3. 100 mg = _____ g   **6.** ¼ gr = _____ mg

Conversion in Metric, Apothecary, and Household Systems by <u>Liquid Volume</u>

LITERS AND OUNCES   1 L = 32 oz

a. To convert liters and quarts to ounces, *multiply* the number of liters by 32, the constant value.
b. To convert ounces to liters or quarts, *divide* the number of ounces by 32, the constant value.

EXAMPLES

PROBLEM 1: Change 3 liters to ounces.

$$3 \text{ L} \times 32 = 96 \text{ oz, or fl } ℥ \text{ (ounces)}$$

PROBLEM 2: Change 64 ounces to liters.

$$64 \text{ oz} \div 32 = 2 \text{ L (liters)}$$

OUNCES AND MILLILITERS   1 oz = 30 mL

a. To convert ounces to milliliters, *multiply* the number of ounces by 30, the constant value.
b. To convert milliliters to ounces, *divide* the number of milliliters by 30, the constant value.

EXAMPLES

PROBLEM 1: Change 5 ounces to milliliters.

$$5 \text{ oz} \times 30 = 150 \text{ mL (milliliters)}$$

PROBLEM 2: Change 120 milliliters to ounces.

$$120 \text{ mL} \div 30 = 4 \text{ oz or fl } ℥ \text{ (ounces)}$$

MILLILITERS AND DROPS   1 mL = 15 drops (gtt) or 15 minims (♏) (number of drops may vary according to the size of the dropper)

a. To convert milliliters to minims or drops, *multiply* the number of milliliters by 15, the constant value.
b. To convert minims and drops to milliliters, *divide* the number of minims or drops by 15, the constant value.

EXAMPLES

PROBLEM 1: Change 4 milliliters to minims and drops.

$$4 \text{ mL} \times 15 = 60 \text{ minims or } 60 \text{ drops}$$

PROBLEM 2: Change 10 drops (gtt) to milliliters.

$$10 \text{ ℳ or gtt} \div 15 = \frac{2}{3} \text{ mL or } 0.667 \text{ mL or } 0.7 \text{ mL}$$

If it is difficult for you to recall these methods, then use the ratio and proportion method to convert from one system to the other.

You must MEMORIZE:

$$30 \text{ mL} = 1 \text{ oz} = 8 \text{ dr} = 2 \text{ T} = 6t$$

These are equivalent values.

Ratio and Proportion The ratio method is useful when converting smaller units within the three systems.

EXAMPLES

PROBLEM 1: Change 20 mL to teaspoons.

	Known			Desired	
mL	:	t	: :	mL	:	t
30	:	6	: :	20	:	X

$$30 \text{ X} = 120$$
$$X = 4 \text{ t (teaspoons)}$$

PROBLEM 2: Change 15 mL to tablespoons.

	Known			Desired	
mL	:	T	: :	mL	:	T
30	:	2	: :	15	:	X

$$30 \text{ X} = 30$$
$$X = 1 \text{ T (tablespoon)}$$

PROBLEM 3: Change 5 oz to tablespoons.

	Known			Desired	
oz	:	T	: :	oz	:	T
1	:	2	: :	5	:	X

$$X = 10 \text{ T (tablespoons)}$$

II. Practice Problems: Conversion by Liquid Volume

Liters and Ounces

1. 2.5 L = _____ oz (fl oz, fl ℥)

2. 0.25 L = _____ oz

3. 40 oz (fl oz, fl ℥) = _____ L

4. 24 oz = _____ L

Ounces and Milliliters

1. 4 oz (fl oz, fl ℥) = _____ mL

2. 6½ oz = _____ mL

3. ½ oz = _____ mL

4. 45 mL = _____ oz

5. 150 mL = _____ oz

6. 15 mL = _____ oz

Milliliters and Drops

1. 1.5 mL = _____ gtt

2. 12 mL = _____ gtt

3. 20 gtt = _____ mL

4. 8 gtt = _____ mL

ANSWERS

I. Conversion by Weight

Grams and Grains

1. 10 × 15 = 150 gr
2. 0.5 × 15 = 7.5 or 7½ gr
3. 0.1 × 15 = 1.5 or 1½ gr

4. 0.03 × 15 = 0.45 or 0.5 gr
5. 3 ÷ 15 = 0.2 g
6. 1.5 ÷ 15 = 0.1 g

Grains and Milligrams

1. 4 × 60 = 240 mg
2. 1.5 × 60 = 90 (100) mg
3. 7.5 × 60 = 450 mg
4. 0.5 × 60 = 30 mg
5. 150 ÷ 60 = 2.5 or 2½ gr

6. 30 ÷ 60 = 0.5 or ½ gr
7. 15 ÷ 60 = ¼ gr
8. 0.6 ÷ 60 =
$$60\overline{)0.60} \overset{.01}{} = 0.01 \text{ or } \tfrac{1}{100} \text{ gr}$$

Ratio and Proportion: Grams, Milligrams, and Grains

1. g : mg : : g : mg
    1 : 1000 : : 2.5 : X
       X = 2500 mg

or

Move decimal point three spaces to the right (conversion within the metric system)

       2.5 g = 2.500 mg ↘↗

2. g : gr : : g : gr
    1 : 15 : : 0.5 : X
       X = 7.5 or 7½ gr

3. mg : g : : mg : g
    1000 : 1 : : 100 : X
       1000 X = 100
          X = 0.1 g

4. mg : g : : mg : g
    1000 : 1 : : 500 : X
       1000 X = 500
          X = 0.5 g

5. g : gr : : g : gr
    1 : 15 : : X : 1
       15 X = 1
          X = 0.06 g

6. gr : mg : : gr : mg
    1 : 60 : : 0.25 : X
       X = 60 × 0.25
       X = 15 mg

II. Conversion by Liquid Volume

Liters and Ounces

1. 2.5 L × 32 = 80 oz
2. 0.25 L × 32 = 8 oz

3. 40 oz ÷ 32 = 1.25 L
4. 24 oz ÷ 32 = 0.75 L

Ounces and Milliliters

1. 4 oz × 30 = 120 mL
2. 6.5 oz × 30 = 195 mL
3. 0.5 oz × 30 = 15 mL

4. 45 mL ÷ 30 = 1½ oz
5. 150 mL ÷ 30 = 5 oz
6. 15 mL ÷ 30 = ½ oz

Milliliters and Drops

1. 1.5 mL × 15 = 22.5 or 23 gtt
2. 12 ℳ × 1 = 12 gtt (1 ℳ = 1 gt)

3. 20 gtt ÷ 15 = 1.3 mL
4. 8 gtt ÷ 15 = 0.5 mL

SUMMARY PRACTICE PROBLEMS

Before computing dosage problems, one system of measurement must be selected. If a medication is ordered in one system and the drug label is in another system, then conversion to one of the systems is necessary. As previously stated, it may be easier to convert to the system used on the drug label.

There are three methods of conversion for the three systems: (1) memorization of a conversion table, (2) conversion methods, and (3) ratio method. You need to convert not only within three systems, but also within the same system if units are not the same, e.g., grams and milligrams. Again, units of measurement *must* be the same to solve problems.

Remember: Multiply when converting from larger to smaller units, and *divide* when converting from smaller to larger units.

Weight: Metric and Apothecary Conversion

1. To convert grams to grains, _____ the number of grams by _____; to convert grains to grams, _____ the number of grains by _____.

    a. 2 g = _____ gr
    b. 7½ gr (gr v̄iīsṡ) = _____ g
    c. 3 gr = _____ g

    d. 0.02 g = _____ gr
    e. 150 gr = _____ g
    f. 0.06 g = _____ gr

2. To convert grains to milligrams, _____ the number of grains by _____; to convert milligrams to grains, _____ the number of milligrams by _____.

    a. 3 gr (gr iīi) = _____ mg
    b. 10 mg = _____ gr
    c. ¼ gr = _____ mg

    d. 5 gr = _____ mg
    e. 7½ gr = _____ mg
    f. 0.4 mg = _____ gr

3. Ratio and proportion

    Remember: 1 g or 1000 mg = 15 gr; 60 (65) mg = 1 gr

    a. Change 5 g to gr

    _____

    b. Change 120 mg to gr

    _____

Volume: Metric, Apothecary, and Household Conversion

4. To convert liters and quarts to ounces, _____ the number of liters by _____; to convert ounces to liters and quarts, _____ the number of ounces by _____.

    a. 3 L = _____ oz (fl ℥)   **d.** ½ L = _____ oz

    b. 1½ qt = _____ oz   **e.** 8 oz = _____ L or qt

    c. 64 oz (fl ℥) = _____ qt   **f.** 24 oz = _____ qt

5. To convert ounces to milliliters, _____ the number of ounces by _____; to convert milliliters to ounces, _____ the number of milliliters by _____.

    a. 1½ oz = _____ mL   **d.** 75 mL = _____ oz (fl ℥)

    b. 15 mL = _____ oz (fl ℥)   **e.** 3 oz (fl ℥) = _____ mL

    c. 60 mL = _____ oz   **f.** 8 oz = _____ mL

6. To convert milliliters to minims or drops, _____ the number of milliliters by _____; to convert minims or drops to milliliters, _____ the number of minims or drops by _____.

    a. 15 mL = _____ ♏ or gtt   **d.** 4 mL = _____ ♏ or gtt

    b. 10 gtt = _____ mL   **e.** 30 ♏ or gtt = _____ mL

    c. 18 ♏ or gtt = _____ mL   **f.** ½ mL = _____ gtt

7. Ratio and proportion
Remember: 30 ml = 1 oz = 8 dr = 2 T = 6 t

    a. Change 16 oz (fl ℥) to L or qt

    b. Change 1½ oz to T

    c. Change 1 T to t

    d. Change 20 mL to t

    e. Change 2½ oz to mL

    f. Change 4 oz to mL

ANSWERS: SUMMARY PRACTICE PROBLEMS

1. multiply, 15; divide, 15

    a. 2 g × 15 = 30 gr   **d.** 0.02 g × 15 = 0.3 or ⅓ gr

    b. 7.5 gr ÷ 15 = ½ or 0.5 g   **e.** 150 gr ÷ 15 = 10 g

    c. 3 gr ÷ 15 = 0.2 g   **f.** 0.06 g × 15 = 0.9 or 1 gr
                                           (round off to 1)

2. multiply, 60; divide, 60

    a. 3 gr × 60 = 180 mg

    b. 10 mg ÷ 60 = $^{10}/_{60}$ = $^{1}/_{6}$ gr

    c. 0.25 gr × 60 = 15 mg

    d. 5 gr × 60 = 300 mg

    e. 7.5 gr × 60 = 450 mg

    f. 0.4 mg ÷ 60 = $^{4}/_{600}$ = $^{1}/_{150}$ gr

3. Ratio and proportion

    a.   *Known*   *Desired*

$$\begin{array}{ccccccc} g & : & gr & :: & g & : & gr \\ 1 & : & 15 & :: & 5 & : & X \end{array}$$
$$X = 75\ gr$$

    b.
$$\begin{array}{ccccccc} gr & : & mg & :: & gr & : & mg \\ 1 & : & 60 & :: & X & : & 120 \end{array}$$
$$60\ X = 120$$
$$X = 2\ gr$$

                or

$$\begin{array}{ccccccc} mg & : & gr & :: & mg & : & gr \\ 60 & : & 1 & :: & 120 & : & X \end{array}$$
$$60\ X = 120$$
$$X = 2\ gr$$

4. multiply, 32; divide, 32

    a. 3 L × 32 = 96 oz

    b. 1.5 qt × 32 = 48 oz

    c. 64 oz ÷ 32 = 2 qt

    d. 0.5 L × 32 = 16 oz

    e. 8 oz ÷ 32 = $^{8}/_{32}$ = $^{1}/_{4}$ L or $^{1}/_{4}$ qt

    f. 24 oz ÷ 32 = $^{24}/_{32}$ = $^{3}/_{4}$ qt

5. multiply, 30; divide, 30

    a. 1½ oz × 30 = 45 mL

    b. 15 mL ÷ 30 = $^{15}/_{30}$ = ½ oz

    c. 60 mL ÷ 30 = 2 oz

    d. 75 mL ÷ 30 = 2½ oz

    e. 3 oz × 30 = 90 mL

    f. 8 oz × 30 = 240 mL

6. multiply, 15; divide, 15

    a. 15 mL × 15 = 225 ℳ or gtt

    b. 10 gtt ÷ 15 = $^{10}/_{15}$ = $^{2}/_{3}$ mL

    c. 18 ℳ or gtt ÷ 15 = 1$^{1}/_{5}$ mL

    d. 4 ml × 15 = 60 ℳ or gtt

    e. 30 ℳ or gtt ÷ 15 = 2 mL

    f. ½ mL × 15 = 7.5 gtt

7. Ratio and proportion

       Known   *Desired*

    a.
$$\begin{array}{ccccccc} L & : & oz & :: & L & : & oz \\ 1 & : & 32 & :: & X & : & 16 \end{array}$$
$$32\ X = 16$$
$$X = \tfrac{1}{2}\ L$$

    b.
$$\begin{array}{ccccccc} oz & : & T & :: & oz & : & T \\ 1 & : & 2 & :: & 1\tfrac{1}{2} & : & X \end{array}$$
$$X = 3\ T$$

    c.
$$\begin{array}{ccccccc} T & : & t & :: & T & : & t \\ 2 & : & 6 & :: & 1 & : & X \end{array}$$
$$2\ X = 6$$
$$X = 3\ t$$

    d.
$$\begin{array}{ccccccc} mL & : & t & :: & mL & : & t \\ 30 & : & 6 & :: & 20 & : & X \end{array}$$
$$30\ X = 120$$
$$X = 4\ t$$

e. oz : mL : : oz : mL
1 : 30 : : 2½ : X
X = 75 mL

f. oz : mL : : oz : mL
1 : 30 : : 4 : X
X = 120 mL

Interpretation of Drug Labels, Drug Orders, Charting, "5 Rights," and Abbreviations

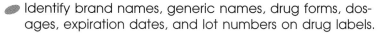

O B J E C T I V E S

- Identify brand names, generic names, drug forms, dosages, expiration dates, and lot numbers on drug labels.
- Give examples of drugs with ``look-alike'' drug names.
- Recognize the components of a drug order.
- Identify the drug information for charting purposes.
- Name the ``5 rights'' in drug administration and give examples of each.
- Utilize the chart related to the ``5 rights.''
- Provide meanings of abbreviations listed in the four categories: drug form, drug measurement, route of drug administration, and times of drug administration.

INTERPRETING DRUG LABELS

The pharmaceutical companies label drugs with their brand name of the drug in large letters and the generic name in smaller letters. The form of the drug (tablet, capsule, liquid, or powder) and dosage are printed on the drug label.

Many of the calculation problems in this book use drug labels. By using drug labels, the student is able to practice solving drug problems that are applicable to clinical practice. The student should know what information is on a drug label and how this information is used in drug calculations. All drug labels provide seven basic items of data: (1) brand name, (2) generic name, (3) dosage, (4) form of the drug, (5) expiration date, (6) lot number, and (7) name of the manufacturer.

EXAMPLE OF DRUG LABEL

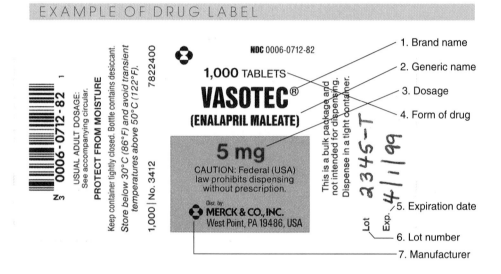

1. **The brand name** is the commercial name given by the pharmaceutical company (manufacturer of the drug). It is printed in large, bold letters.

2. **The generic name** is the chemical name given to the drug, regardless of the drug manufacturer. It is printed in smaller letters, usually under the brand name.

3. **The dosage** is the drug dose per drug form (tablet, capsule, liquid) as stated on the label.

4. **The form of the drug** (tablet, capsule, liquid) relates to the dosage.

5. **The expiration date** refers to the length of time the drug can be used before losing its potency. Drugs should not be administered after the expiration date. The nurse must check the expiration date of all drugs he or she administers.

6. **The lot number** identifies the drug batch in which the medication was produced. Occasionally, a drug is recalled according to the lot number.

7. **The manufacturer** is the pharmaceutical company that produces the brand name drug.

Examples of drug labels are given, and practice problems for reading drug labels follow the examples.

EXAMPLE 1: ORAL DRUG (SOLID FORM)

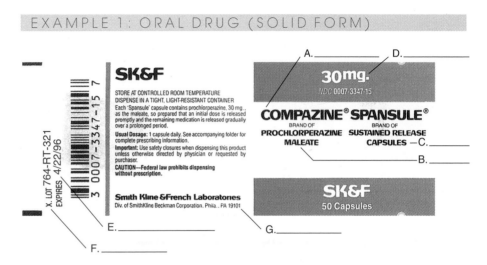

a. Brand name is Compazine

b. Generic name is prochlorperazine

c. Drug form is a sustained release capsule (SR capsule)

d. Dosage is 30 mg per capsule

e. Expiration date is 4/22/96 (after this date, the drug should be discarded)

f. Lot number is 764-RT-321

g. Manufacturer is Smith Kline & French Laboratories

EXAMPLE 2: ORAL DRUG (LIQUID FORM)

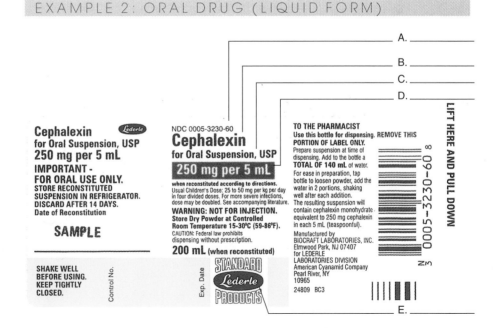

a. Brand name is none (Manufactored as a generic drug)

b. Generic name is cephalexin

c. Drug form is oral suspension

d. Dosage is 250 mg per 5 mL

e. Manufacturer is Lederle.

EXAMPLE 3: INJECTABLE DRUG

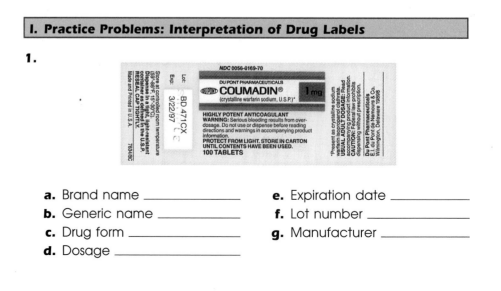

F. _____

E. _____

A. _____

B. _____

C. _____

D. _____

a. Brand name is Mandol

b. Generic name is cefamandole nafate

c. Drug form is drug powder that must be reconstituted in a liquid form for use

d. Dosage is 500 mg drug powder

e. Drug container is vial

f. IV: reconstitute by using at least 5 mL of sterile water for injection which then must be diluted in 50 to 100 mL of IV fluids.
IM: 2 mL of a diluent should be added. The total amount of the drug would then equal 2.2 mL. The powder increases the liquid form by 0.2 mL.

I. Practice Problems: Interpretation of Drug Labels

1.

a. Brand name _____

b. Generic name _____

c. Drug form _____

d. Dosage _____

e. Expiration date _____

f. Lot number _____

g. Manufacturer _____

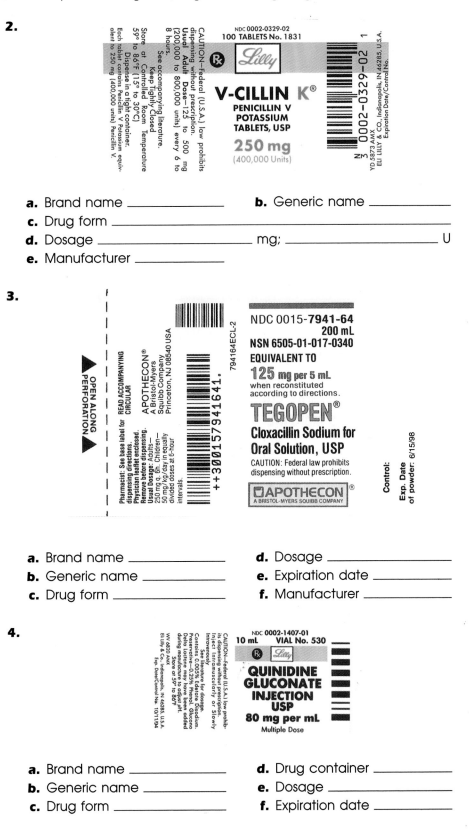

2.

NDC 0002-0329-02
100 TABLETS No. 1831

Lilly

V-CILLIN K®
PENICILLIN V
POTASSIUM
TABLETS, USP

250 mg
(400,000 Units)

CAUTION—Federal (U.S.A.) law prohibits dispensing without prescription.
Usual Adult Dose—125 to 500 mg (200,000 to 800,000 units) every 6 to 8 hours.

See accompanying literature.
Keep Tightly Closed
Store at Controlled Room Temperature 59° to 86°F (15° to 30°C)
Dispense in a tight container.
Each tablet contains Penicillin V Potassium equivalent to 250 mg (400,000 units) Penicillin V.

N3 0002-0329-02 1
YD 5873 AMX
ELI LILLY & CO., Indianapolis, IN 46285, U.S.A.
Expiration Date/Control No.

a. Brand name _____   **b.** Generic name _____
c. Drug form _____
d. Dosage _____ mg; _____ U
e. Manufacturer _____

3.

OPEN ALONG PERFORATION

READ ACCOMPANYING CIRCULAR
APOTHECON®
A Bristol-Myers
Squibb Company
Princeton, NJ 08540 USA

79416ECL-2

Pharmacist: See base label for dispensing directions.
Physician leaflet enclosed.
Remove before dispensing.
Usual Dosage: Adults—250 mg q. 6h. Children—50 mg/kg/day in equally divided doses at 6-hour intervals.

+ +300157941641.

NDC 0015-**7941-64**
200 mL
NSN 6505-01-017-0340
EQUIVALENT TO
125 mg per 5 mL
when reconstituted
according to directions.

TEGOPEN®
**Cloxacillin Sodium for
Oral Solution, USP**
CAUTION: Federal law prohibits
dispensing without prescription.

☐**APOTHECON**®
A BRISTOL-MYERS SQUIBB COMPANY

Control:
Exp. Date
of powder: 6/15/98

a. Brand name _____   **d.** Dosage _____
b. Generic name _____   **e.** Expiration date _____
c. Drug form _____   **f.** Manufacturer _____

4.

NDC 0002-1407-01
10 mL   VIAL No. 530

Ⓡ *Lilly*

**QUINIDINE
GLUCONATE
INJECTION
USP**
80 mg per mL
Multiple Dose

CAUTION—Federal (U.S.A.) law prohibits dispensing without prescription.
Inject Intramuscularly or Slowly Intravenously
See literature for dosage.
Contains 0.005% Edetate Disodium. Preservative—0.25% Phenol. Gluconic Delta Lactone may have been added during manufacture to adjust pH.
Store at 59° to 86°F
WV 6820 AMX
ELI LILLY & Co., Indianapolis, IN 46285, U.S.A.
Exp. Date/Control No. 10/11/94

a. Brand name _____   **d.** Drug container _____
b. Generic name _____   **e.** Dosage _____
c. Drug form _____   **f.** Expiration date _____

5.

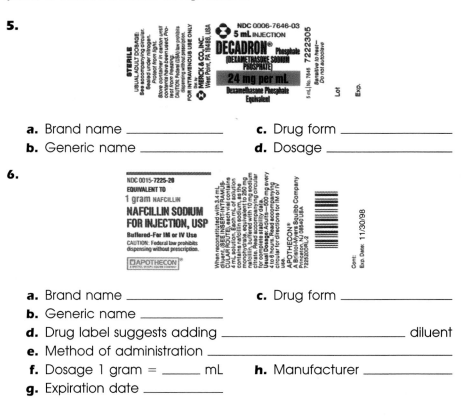

NDC 0006-7646-03
5 mL INJECTION
DECADRON® Phosphate
(DEXAMETHASONE SODIUM PHOSPHATE)
24 mg per mL
Dexamethasone Phosphate Equivalent

STERILE
USUAL ADULT DOSAGE.
See accompanying circular.
Sealed under nitrogen.
Protect from light.
Store container in carton until contents have been used. Protect from freezing.
CAUTION: Federal (USA) law prohibits dispensing without prescription.
FOR INTRAVENOUS USE ONLY

Dist. by
MERCK & CO., INC.
West Point, PA 19486, USA

7222305

5 mL No. 7646

Sensitive to heat—
Do not autoclave

Lot

Exp.

a. Brand name _____   **c.** Drug form _____

b. Generic name _____   **d.** Dosage _____

6.

NDC 0015-7225-20
EQUIVALENT TO
1 gram NAFCILLIN
NAFCILLIN SODIUM
FOR INJECTION, USP
Buffered-For IM or IV Use
CAUTION: Federal law prohibits dispensing without prescription.
☐ APOTHECON®
A BRISTOL-MYERS SQUIBB COMPANY

When reconstituted with 3.4 mL diluent, (SEE INSERT: INTRAMUS-CULAR ROUTE), each vial contains 4 mL solution. Each mL of solution contains nafcillin sodium, as the monohydrate, equivalent to 250 mg nafcillin, buffered with 10 mg sodium citrate. Read accompanying circular for complete stability data.
Usual Dosage: Adults—500 mg every 4 to 6 hours. Read accompanying circular for directions for IM or IV use.

APOTHECON®
A Bristol-Myers Squibb Company
Princeton, NJ 08540 USA
7225DRL-2

Cont:
Exp. Date: 11/30/98

a. Brand name _____   **c.** Drug form _____

b. Generic name _____

d. Drug label suggests adding _____ diluent

e. Method of administration _____

f. Dosage 1 gram = _____ mL   **h.** Manufacturer _____

g. Expiration date _____

DRUG DIFFERENTIATION

Some drugs with similar names, such as quinine and quinidine, have different chemical drug structures. Extreme care must be exercised when administering drugs that ''look alike'' or that have similar spellings.

Percocet contains oxycodone and acetaminophen, whereas Percodan contains oxycodone and aspirin. A patient may be allergic to aspirin or should not take aspirin; therefore, it is important that the patient is given Percocet. *Read the drug labels carefully.*

EXAMPLES: PERCOCET AND PERCODAN

NDC 0060-0127-70   NSN 6505-01-082-5509

DU PONT PHARMACEUTICALS
(DUPONT) **PERCOCET®**
(oxycodone and acetaminophen tablets, USP)

Each tablet contains:
Oxycodone hydrochloride . . . . 5 mg*
WARNING: May be habit forming
Acetaminophen, USP . . . . 325 mg
*5 mg oxycodone HCl is equivalent to 4.4815 mg of oxycodone.

CAUTION: Federal law prohibits dispensing without prescription.
DOSAGE: For dosage and full prescribing information, read accompanying product information.
DEA ORDER FORM REQUIRED

100 TABLETS

Store at controlled room temperature (15°-30°C, 59°-86°F). Dispense in a tight, light-resistant container as defined in the USP.

Lot:
Exp:
SAMPLE

Du Pont Pharmaceuticals Caribe, Inc.
Subsidiary of E.I. du Pont de Nemours & Co.
P.O. Box 12, Manati, Puerto Rico 00701

7443/BK

0060-0127-70

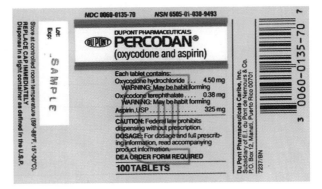

Drug Orders

Medication orders may be prescribed and written by a physician (MD), osteopathic physician (DO), dentist (DDS), podiatrist (DPM), or a licensed health care provider who has been given authority by the state to write prescriptions. Drug prescriptions in private practice or in clinics are written on a small prescription pad and filled by a pharmacist at a drug store or hospital (see Figure 3–1). For hospitalized patients, the drug orders are written on a doctor's order sheet and signed by the physician or licensed health provider (see Figure 3–2). If the order is given by telephone (TO), the order must be cosigned by the physician in 24 hours. Most health institutions have policies concerning verbal or telephone drug orders. The nurse must know and must follow the institution's policy.

PRESCRIPTION PAD MEDICATION ORDER

```
                    Roger J. Smith, Jr., M.D.
                         678 Apple Street
                   Wilmington, Delaware 19810
 (123) 456-7891
 ────────────────────────────────────────────────────
 NAME _____  Age _____
 Address _____   Date _____

 Rx


 Label_____          _____ M.D.
 Safety Cap_____
 Refill _____ times
```

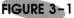

FIGURE 3–1

PATIENT'S ORDERS

CITY HOSPITAL Dover, Delaware	PATIENT'S NAME Room #	
Date	Time	Patient's Orders

FIGURE 3–2

The basic components of a drug order include (1) date and time the order was written, (2) drug name, (3) drug dosage, (4) route of administration, (5) frequency of administration, and (6) physician or health care provider's signature. It is the nurse's responsibility to follow the physician's order, but if any one of these components is missing, the drug order is incomplete and cannot be carried out. If the order is illegible, is missing a component, or calls for an inappropriate drug or dosage, clarification must be obtained before the order is carried out.

Examples of drug orders and their interpretation are:

6/3/97   9:10A   Digoxin 0.25 mg, po, qd
                         (give 0.25 mg of digoxin by mouth daily)
───
                         Ibuprofen 400 mg, po, q4h, PRN
                         (give 400 mg of ibuprofen by mouth every 4 hours as needed)
───
                         Cefadyl 500 mg, IM, q6h
                         (give 500 mg of Cefadyl intramuscularly every 6 hours)
───
                         Prednisone 5 mg, po, q8h × 5 days
                         (give 5 mg of prednisone by mouth every 8 hours for 5 days)
───

II. Practice Problems: Interpretation of Drug Orders

Interpret these drug orders. For abbreviations that are unknown, see the section on abbreviations later in this chapter.

1. Tetracycline 250 mg, po, q6h

_____

2. HydroDIURIL 50 mg, po, qd

_____

3. Meperidine 50 mg, IM, q3-4h, PRN

_____

4. Ancef 1 g, IV, q8h

_____

5. Prednisone 10 mg, tid × 5 days

_____

List what is missing in these drug orders.

6. Codeine 30 mg, po, PRN for pain _____

7. Digoxin 0.25 mg, qd _____

8. Ceclor 125 mg, po _____

9. TheoDur 200 mg _____

10. Penicillin V K 200,000 U, for days _____

_____

There are four types of drug orders: (1) standing order, (2) one-time (single) order, (3) PRN (whenever necessary) order, and (4) STAT (immediately) order (Table 3–1). Many of the drugs ordered for nonhospitalized patients are normally

TABLE 3–1
Types of Drug Orders

TYPES/DESCRIPTION	EXAMPLES
Standing orders: A standing order may be typed or written on the doctor's order sheet. It may be an order that is given for a number of days, or it may be a routine order for all patients who had the same type of procedure. Standing orders may include PRN orders.	Erythromycin 250 mg, po, q6h, 5 days Demerol 50 mg, IM, q3–4h, PRN, pain Colace 100 mg, po, hs, PRN

One-time (single) orders:
    One-time orders are given once, usually at a specified time
	Preoperative orders:
	    Meperidine 75 mg, IM, 7:30 AM
	    Atropine SO$_4$ 0.4 mg, IM, 7:30 AM

PRN orders: PRN orders are given at the patient's request and at the nurse's judgment concerning safety and need	Pentobarbital 100 mg, hs, PRN Darvocet-N, tab 1, q4h, PRN
STAT orders: A STAT order is for a one-time drug given immediately	Regular Insulin 10 U, SC, STAT

standing orders that can be renewed (refilled) for 6 months. Narcotics are *not* automatically refilled; if the narcotic usage is extended, the physician writes another prescription or calls the pharmacy.

Charting Medications

Charting on medication records should be done immediately after giving the medications. Delay in charting could result in (1) forgetting to chart the drugs, or (2) administration of the drugs by another nurse who thought the drugs were *not* given.

Medication records (charts) differ among health care facilities. Drug information that should be on the medication record includes (1) date drug was ordered, (2) drug name, (3) dosage, (4) route of administration, (5) frequency of administration,

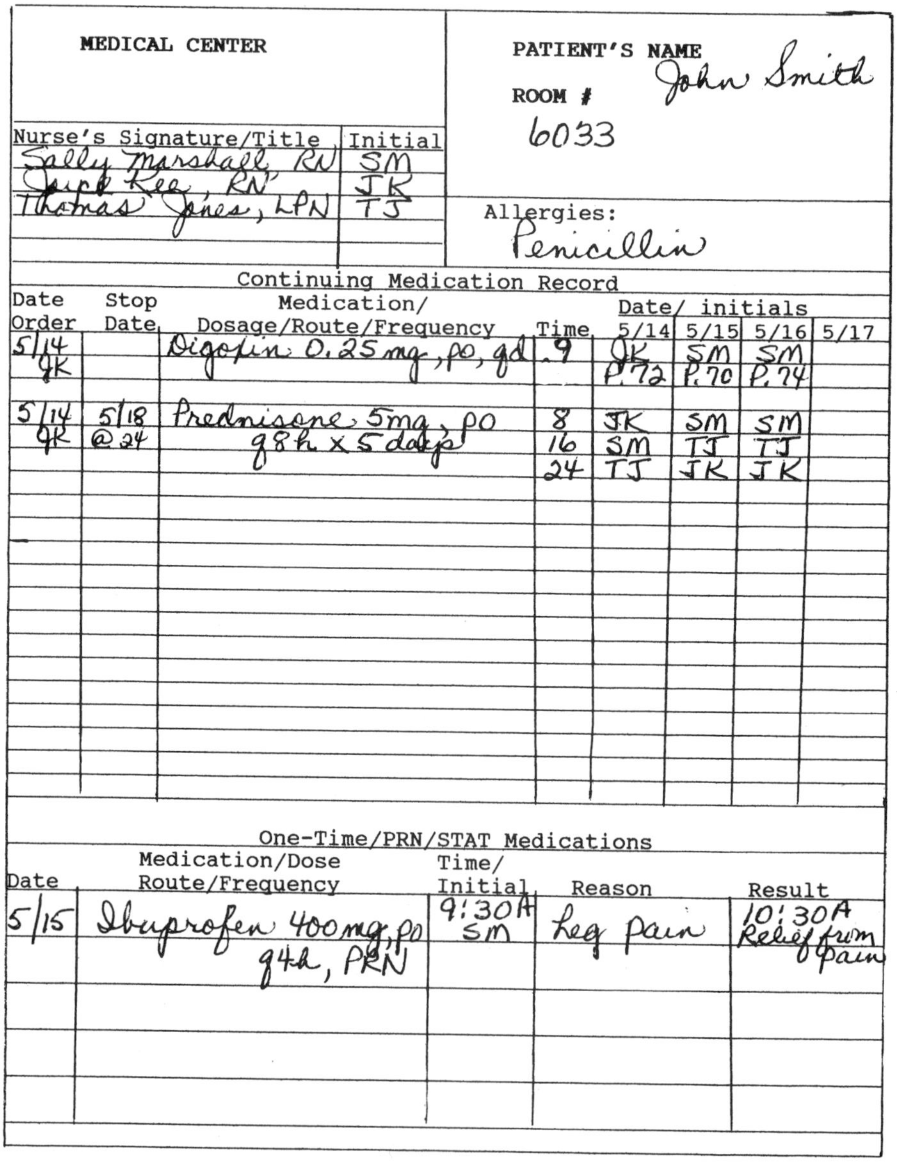

MEDICAL CENTER		PATIENT'S NAME			John Smith
		ROOM # 6033			
Nurse's Signature/Title	**Initial**				
Sally Marshall, RN	SM				
Jack Lee, RN	JK	Allergies:			
Thomas Jones, LPN	TJ	Penicillin			

Continuing Medication Record

Date Order	Stop Date	Medication/ Dosage/Route/Frequency	Time	Date/ initials 5/14	5/15	5/16	5/17
5/14 JK		Digoxin 0.25 mg, po, qd	9	JK P.72	SM P.70	SM P.74	
5/14 JK	5/18 @24	Prednisone 5mg, po q8h x 5 days	8	JK	SM	SM	
			16	SM	TJ	TJ	
			24	TJ	JK	JK	

One-Time/PRN/STAT Medications

Date	Medication/Dose Route/Frequency	Time/ Initial	Reason	Result
5/15	Ibuprofen 400mg, po q4h, PRN	9:30A SM	Leg pain	10:30A Relief from pain

FIGURE 3-3

(6) date and time drug was given, and (7) nurse's signature and initials. An example of a medication record is illustrated in Figure 3–3.

Methods of Drug Distribution

Two methods of drug distribution frequently used for administering medications are the stock drug method and the unit dose method. Table 3–2 describes these methods and lists the advantages and disadvantages of each.

THE "5 RIGHTS" IN DRUG ADMINISTRATION

To provide safe drug administration, the nurse should practice the "5 rights": the right client, the right drug, the right dose, the right time, and the right route. Three additional rights could be added: the right documentation, the right of the client to know the reason for administration of the drug, and the right of the client to refuse to take a medication.

RIGHT CLIENT: Checking the client's identification band should always take place before giving a medication to the client.

- 🖉 Verify client by checking his or her identification bracelet.
- 🖉 Ask the client his or her name. Do not call the client by name. Some individuals answer to any name.
- 🖉 Check the name on the client's medication label.

RIGHT DRUG: To avoid error, the nurse should:

- 🖉 Check the drug label 3 times: (1) with first contact with the drug bottle, (2) before pouring the drug, and (3) after pouring the drug.

TABLE 3-2
Methods of Drug Distribution

	STOCK DRUG METHOD	UNIT DOSE METHOD
Description	Drug is stored in large containers on the floor and is dispensed from the container for all patients	Drug is packaged in single doses by the pharmacy for 24-hour dosing
Advantages	Drug is always available, which eliminates time spent waiting for drug to arrive from the pharmacy Cost efficiency is enhanced by having large quantities of the drug	Packaging saves the nurse time otherwise spent in preparing the drug dose Correct dose is provided with *no* calculation needed Drug is billed for specific number of doses
Disadvantages	Drug error is more prevalent because the drug is "poured" by many persons More drugs to choose from, which may cause error Drug expiration date on the container may be missed	There is time delay in receiving the drug from pharmacy If the doses are contaminated or damaged, they are not immediately replaceable

- Check that the drug order is complete and legible. If it is not, contact the physician or charge nurse.
- Know the drug action.
- Check the expiration date. Discard an outdated drug or return the drug to the pharmacy.
- If client questions the drug, recheck drug and drug dose. If in doubt, seek another health care personnel's advice, e.g., pharmacist, physician, licensed health care provider. Some generic drugs have a different shape or color.

RIGHT DOSE: Stock drugs and unit dose drugs are the two methods frequently used for drug distribution. Not all health care institutions use the unit dose method (drugs prepared by dose in the pharmacy or by the pharmaceutical company). If the institution uses the unit dose method, drugs in bottles should *not* be administered without the consent of the physician or pharmacist.

- Be able to calculate drug dose using the ratio and proportion, basic formula, or dimensional analysis method
- Know how to calculate drug dose by body weight (kg) or by body surface area (BSA; m²). Drug doses for potent drugs (e.g., anticancer agents) and for children frequently use body weight or BSA to determine the drug dose.
- Know the recommended dosage range for the drug. Check the *Physician's Desk Reference*, the *American Hospital Formulary*, or another drug reference. If the nurse feels the dose is incorrect or not within the therapeutic range, he or she should notify the charge nurse, physician, or pharmacist, and document all communications.
- Recalculate drug dose if in doubt, or have a colleague recheck the dose.
- Question drug doses that appear to be incorrect.
- Have a colleague check the drug dose of potent or specified drugs such as insulin, digoxin, narcotics, and anticancer agents. This procedure is required by some facilities.

RIGHT TIME: The drug dose should be given at a specified time to maintain a therapeutic drug serum level. Too-frequent dosing can cause drug toxicity, and missed doses can nullify the drug action and its effect.

- Administer the drug at the specified time(s). Drugs can be given ½ hour before or after the time prescribed.
- Omit or delay a drug dose according to specific circumstance, i.e., laboratory and diagnostic tests. Notify the appropriate personnel of the reason.
- Administer drugs that are affected by foods, e.g., tetracycline, 1 hour before or 2 hours after meals.
- Administer drugs that can irritate the gastric mucosa, e.g., potassium or aspirin, with foods.

CHECKLIST FOR THE "5 RIGHTS" IN DRUG ADMINISTRATION

Right Client

- 🔹 Check client's identification bracelet. ☐
- 🔹 Ask the client for his or her name. ☐
- 🔹 Check the name on the client's medication label. ☐

Right Drug

- 🔹 Check that the drug order is complete and legible. ☐
- 🔹 Check the drug label 3 times. ☐
- 🔹 Check the expiration date. ☐
- 🔹 Know the drug action. ☐

Right Dose

- 🔹 Calculate the drug dose. ☐
- 🔹 Know the recommended dosage range for the drug. ☐
- 🔹 Recalculate the drug dose with another nurse if in doubt. ☐

Right Time

- 🔹 Administer drug at the specified time(s). ☐
- 🔹 Document any delay or omitted drug dose. ☐
- 🔹 Administer drugs that irritate gastric mucosa with food. ☐
- 🔹 Administer antibiotics at even intervals (q6h, q8h). ☐

Right Route

- 🔹 Know the route for administration of the drug. ☐
- 🔹 Use aseptic techniques when administering a drug. ☐
- 🔹 Document the injection site on the patient's chart. ☐

🔹 Know that drugs with a long half-life ($t_{1/2}$), e.g., 20 to 36 hours, are usually given once per day. Drugs having a short half-life, e.g., 1 to 6 hours, are given several times a day.

🔹 Administer antibiotics at even intervals (e.g., q8h (8-4-12) rather than tid (8-12-4); q6h (6-12-6-12) rather than qid (8-12-4-8)) to maintain a therapeutic drug serum level.

RIGHT ROUTE: The right route is necessary for appropriate absorption of the medication. The more common routes of absorption include (1) oral (by mouth, PO) tablet, capsule, pill, liquid, suspension; (2) sublingual (under the tongue for venous absorption, *not* to be swallowed); (3) buccal (between gum and cheek); (4) topical (applied to the skin); (5) inhalation (aerosol sprays); (6) instillation (in nose, eye, ear, rectum, or vagina); (7) and four parenteral routes: intradermal, subcutaneous, intramuscular, and intravenous.

● Know the drug route. If in doubt, check with the pharmacy. Ointment for the eye should have ''ophthalmic'' written on the tube. Drugs given sublingually (e.g., nitroglycerin tablet) should *not* be swallowed, because the effect of the drug would be lost.

● Administer injectables (subcutaneous and intramuscular) to appropriate sites (see Chap. 7).

● Use aseptic technique when administering drugs. Sterile technique is required with the parenteral routes.

● Document the injection site used on the client's chart or on another designated sheet.

ABBREVIATIONS

Selected abbreviations are listed in four categories: drug form, drug measurements, route of drug administration, and times of drug administration. These abbreviations are frequently used in drug therapy and in this text; therefore, nurses must know the meanings of these abbreviations.

A. Drug Form

ABBREVIATION	MEANING	ABBREVIATION	MEANING
aq	Water	SR	Sustained release
cap	Capsule	supp	Suppository
elix	Elixir	susp	Suspension
emuls	Emulsion	syr	Syrup
ext	Extract	tab	Tablet
mixt	Mixture	tr, tinct	Tincture
		ung	Ointment

B. Drug Measurements

ABBREVIATION	MEANING	ABBREVIATION	MEANING
cc	Cubic centimeter	mL	Milliliter
dL	Deciliter (one-tenth of a liter)	ℳ, min	minim
		ng	Nanogram
dr	Dram	oz	Ounce
fl dr	Fluid dram (fl ʒ)	pt	Pint
fl oz	Fluid ounce (fl ℥)	qt	Quart
g, gm, G, Gm	Gram	ss	One-half
gr	Grain	T.O.	Telephone order
gtt	Drops	T, tbsp	Tablespoon
kg	Kilogram	t, tsp	Teaspoon
l, L	Liter	U	Unit
m², M²	Square meter	V.O.	Verbal order
mcg, μg	Microgram	×	Times
mEq	Milliequivalent	>	Greater than
mg	Milligram	<	Less than

C. Route of Drug Administration

ABBREVIATION	MEANING	ABBREVIATION	MEANING
A.D., ad	Right ear	NGT	Nasogastric tube
A.S., as, al	Left ear	O.D., od	Right eye
A.U., au	Both ears	O.S., os, ol	Left eye
ID	Intradermal	O.U., ou	Both eyes
IM	Intramuscular	P.O., po, os	By mouth
IV	Intravenous	Ⓡ	Right
IVPB	Intravenous piggyback	Rect	Rectal
		SC, subc, sc	Subcutaneous
KVO	Keep vein open	Sl, sl, subl	Sublingual
Ⓛ	Left	Vag	Vaginal

D. Times of Drug Administration

ABBREVIATION	MEANING	ABBREVIATION	MEANING
A.C., ac	Before meals	qd, od	Every day
ad lib	As desired	qh	Every hour
B.i.d., Bid, bid	Twice a day	q2h	Every 2 hours
c̄	With	q4h	Every 4 hours
h	Hour	q6h	Every 6 hours
hs	Hour of sleep	q8h	Every 8 hours
noct	At night	Q.i.d., Qid, qid	Four times a day
NPO	Nothing by mouth	Qod, qod	Every other day
P.C., pc	After meals	s̄	Without
per	By	SOS	Once if necessary, if there is a need
PRN	Whenever necessary, as needed	STAT	Give immediately
q	Every	T.i.d., Tid, tid	Three times a day
qAM	Every morning, every AM		

III. Practice Problems: Abbreviations

If you have more than two incorrect answers, return to abbreviations and meanings and review. Then quiz yourself on the abbreviations.

1. cap _____

2. SR _____

3. fl oz _____

4. g, G _____

5. gr _____

6. L _____

7. mL _____

8. mcg, μg _____

9. mg _____

10. s̄s̄ _____

11. T _____

12. t _____

13. > _____

14. A.U., au _____

15. IM _____

16. IV _____

17. KVO _____

18. O.S. _____

19. O.U. _____   **25.** P.C., pc _____

20. SC _____   **26.** q4h _____

21. c̄ _____   **27.** Qid, qid _____

22. A.C., ac _____   **28.** Tid, tid _____

23. hs _____   **29.** Bid, bid _____

24. NPO _____   **30.** STAT _____

ANSWERS

I. Interpretation of Drug Labels

1. a. Coumadin   **b.** warfarin sodium (crystalline)   **c.** tablet
   d. 1 mg per tablet   **e.** 3/22/97   **f.** BD471CX
   g. Dupont Pharmaceuticals

2. a. V-Cillin K   **b.** penicillin V potassium   **c.** tablet
   d. 250 mg per tablet; 400,000 U per tablet   **e.** Lilly

3. a. Tegopen   **b.** cloxacillin sodium   **c.** liquid for oral administration
   d. 125 mg per 5 ml   **e.** 6/15/98   **f.** Apothecon

4. a. quinidine gluconate
   b. quinidine gluconate (same as brand name)
   c. liquid for injection
   d. vial (multiple dose vial), total amount is 10 mL per vial
   e. 80 mg per mL
   f. 10/11/94 (date expired, do *not* use, return to pharmacy)

5. a. Decadron phosphate   **b.** dexamethasone sodium phosphate
   c. liquid for injection   **d.** 24 mg per mL

6. a. nafcillin sodium   **b.** nafcillin sodium (same as brand name)
   c. drug powder to be reconstituted   **d.** 3.4 mL diluent   **e.** IM or IV
   f. 1 gram = 4 mL   **g.** 11/30/98   **h.** Apothecon

II. Interpretation of Drug Orders

1. Give 250 mg of tetracycline by mouth every 6 hours.

2. Give 50 mg of HydroDIURIL by mouth every day.

3. Give 50 mg of meperidine intramuscularly every 3 to 4 hours whenever necessary.

4. Give 1 g of Ancef intravenously every 8 hours.

5. Give 10 mg of prednisone three times a day for 5 days.

6. frequency of administration

7. route of administration

8. frequency of administration

9. route and frequency of administration

10. route and frequency of administration and stop date

III. Abbreviations

1. capsule   **5.** grain
2. sustained release   **6.** liter
3. fluid ounce   **7.** milliliter
4. gram   **8.** microgram

9. milligram
10. one-half
11. tablespoon
12. teaspoon
13. greater than
14. both ears
15. intramuscular
16. intravenous
17. keep vein open
18. left eye
19. both eyes
20. subcutaneous
21. with
22. before meals
23. hour of sleep
24. nothing by mouth
25. after meals
26. every four hours
27. four times a day
28. three times a day
29. two times a day
30. immediately

CHAPTER

Alternative Methods for Drug Administration

OBJECTIVES

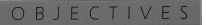

- Recognize the various methods of drug administration.
- Explain the steps (methods) in drug administration using the various methods.

TRANSDERMAL PATCH

INHALATION
Metered-Dose Inhaler
Nasal Inhaler

NASAL SPRAY AND DROPS

EYE DROPS AND OINTMENT

EAR DROPS

PHARYNGEAL SPRAY, MOUTHWASH, AND LOZENGE

TOPICAL PREPARATIONS: LOTION, CREAM, AND OINTMENT

RECTAL SUPPOSITORY

VAGINAL SUPPOSITORY, CREAM, AND OINTMENT

There are numerous methods for administering medications in addition to oral (tablets, capsules, liquid) and parenteral (subcutaneous, intramuscular, intravenous) routes. Alternative methods for drug administration include transdermal patches; inhalation sprays; nasal sprays and drops; eye drops and ointments; ear drops; pharyngeal (throat) sprays, mouthwashes, and lozenges; topical lotions, creams, and ointments; rectal suppositories; and vaginal suppositories, creams, and ointments.

TRANSDERMAL PATCH

PURPOSE: The transdermal patch (Fig. 4–1) contains medication; the patch is applied to the skin for slow, systemic absorption, usually over 24 hours. Use of the transdermal route avoids the gastrointestinal problems associated with some oral medications and provides a more consistent drug level in the patient's blood.

METHOD:

- 🍂 Cleanse the skin area where the patch will be applied. These areas can include the chest, abdomen, arms, or thighs. Avoid areas that have hair.
- 🍂 Remove the transparent cover (inside) of the patch. Do *not* touch the inside of the patch.
- 🍂 Apply the patch to the chosen area with the dull, plastic side up.

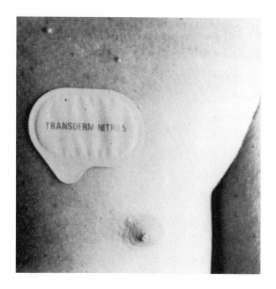

FIGURE 4–1
Transderm-Nitro transdermal patch.
(Courtesy of Ciba-Geigy Pharmaceuticals, Summit, NJ.)

INHALATION

PURPOSE: The drug inhaler delivers the prescribed dose to be absorbed by the mucosal lining of the respiratory tract. The drug categories for respiratory inhalation are bronchodilators, which dilate bronchial tubes; glucocorticoids, which are antiinflammatory agents; and mucolytics, which liquefy bronchial secretions.

METHOD:

Two types of inhalers are the metered-dose inhaler or nebulizer and the nasal inhaler.

Metered-Dose Inhaler

- Insert the medication canister into the plastic holder.
- Shake the inhaler well before using. Remove cap from mouthpiece.
- Instruct the patient to breathe out through the mouth, expelling air. Place the mouthpiece into the patient's mouth, holding the inhaler upright (Fig. 4–2).
- Instruct the patient to keep his or her lips securely around the mouthpiece and inhale. While the patient is inhaling, push the top of the medication canister once.
- Instruct the patient to hold his or her breath for a few seconds, remove the mouthpiece and take your finger off the canister, and tell the patient to exhale slowly.

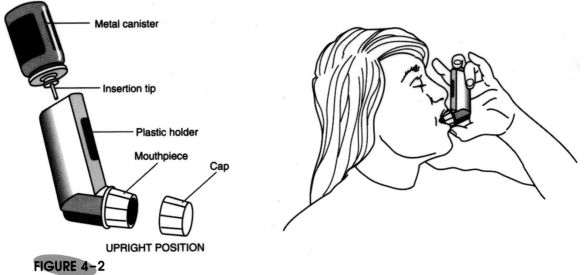

Metal canister

Insertion tip

Plastic holder

Mouthpiece

Cap

UPRIGHT POSITION

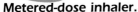

FIGURE 4–2
Metered-dose inhaler.
(Kee J, Hayes E: *Pharmacology: A Nursing Process Approach,* 1993, p 367. Philadelphia, WB Saunders Co.)

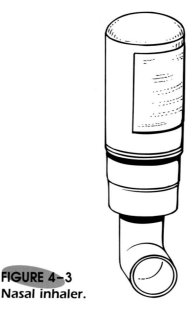

FIGURE 4–3
Nasal inhaler.

● If a second dose is required, wait 1 to 2 minutes and repeat the procedure.

● Cleanse the mouthpiece. If the inhaler has not been used recently or if it is being used for the first time, test spray before administering the metered dose.

Nasal Inhaler

● Instruct the client to blow his or her nose to clear the nostrils.

● Insert the drug cartridge into the adapter (Fig. 4–3).

● Shake the inhaler well before using. Remove the cap.

● Place your finger on top of cartridge.

● Instruct the client to tilt his or her head back slightly. Place the tip of the adapter in one nostril; occlude the other nostril, and have client inhale while pressing the adapter. Inform the client to exhale through his or her mouth.

● Repeat the procedure with the other nostril if ordered.

● Cleanse the tip of the adapter and dry thoroughly.

NASAL SPRAY AND DROPS

PURPOSE: Most drugs in nasal spray and drop containers are to relieve nasal congestion due to upper respiratory infection and polyps by shrinking swollen nasal membranes. Types of drugs given by this method are vasoconstrictors and gluco-corticoids.

METHOD:

Nasal Spray:

● Instruct the client to sit with his or her head tilted slightly back or slightly forward, according to the directions on the spray container (Fig. 4–4).

● Insert the tip of the container in one nostril and occlude the other nostril.

● Instruct the client to inhale as the drug spray container is squeezed. Repeat with the same nostril if ordered.

● Repeat the procedure with the other nostril if ordered.

● Encourage the client to keep his or her head tilted for several minutes until the drug action is effective. The nose should not be blown until the head is upright.

Nose Drops:

● Place the client in an upright position with his or her head tilted back.

● Insert the dropper into the nostril without touching the nasal membranes.

● Instill 2 drops of medications or the amount as prescribed.

● Instruct the client to keep his or her head back for 5 minutes and to breathe through the mouth.

● Cleanse the dropper.

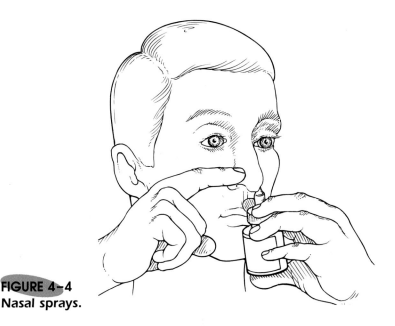

FIGURE 4–4
Nasal sprays.

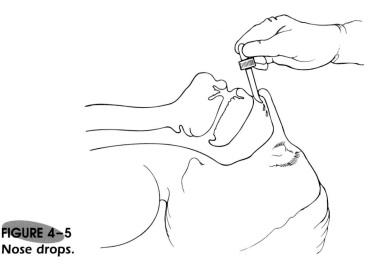

FIGURE 4-5
Nose drops.

🔅 For the medication to reach the sinuses, the client should be in the supine position with head turned to one side and then the other so the medication can reach the frontal and maxillary sinuses. For the ethmoidal and sphenoidal sinuses, the patient's head is lowered below his or her shoulders (Fig. 4-5).

EYE DROPS AND OINTMENT

PURPOSE: Eye medications are prescribed for various eye disorders such as glaucoma, infection, and allergies, and for eye examination and eye surgery.

METHOD:

Eye Drops:

🔅 Instruct the client to lie or sit with his or her head tilted back.

🔅 Instruct the client to look up toward the ceiling and away from the dropper. Pull down the lower lid of the affected eye (Fig. 4–6). Place one drop of medication into the lower conjunctival sac. This prevents the drug from dropping onto the cornea.

🔅 Press gently on the medial nasolacrimal canthus (side closest to the nose) with a tissue to prevent systemic drug absorption.

🔅 If the other eye is affected, repeat the procedure in the other eye.

🔅 Inform the client to blink one or two times and then keep the eyes closed for several minutes. Use a tissue to blot away excess drug fluid.

Eye Ointment:

🔅 Instruct the client to lie or sit with his or her head tilted back.

🔅 Pull down the lower lid to expose the conjunctival sac of the affected eye (Fig. 4–7).

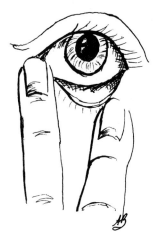

FIGURE 4-6
Eye drops.
(Kee J, Hayes E: *Pharmacology: A Nursing Process Approach,*
1993, p 469. Philadelphia, WB Saunders Co.)

● Squeeze a strip of ointment about ¼ inch long (unless otherwise indicated) onto the conjunctival sac. Medication placed directly
  onto the cornea can cause discomfort or damage.
● If the other eye is affected, repeat the procedure.
● Instruct the client to close his or her eyes for 2 to 3 minutes. Blurred
  vision may occur for a short period of time.

EAR DROPS

PURPOSE: Ear medication is frequently prescribed to soften and loosen the ceru-
men (wax) in the ear canal, for anesthetic effect, to immobilize insects in the ear
canal, and for infection, such as fungal infection.

METHOD:

● Instruct the client to lie on the unaffected side or to sit upright with
  his or her head tilted toward the unaffected side.

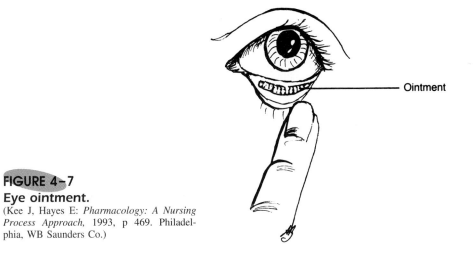

Ointment

FIGURE 4-7
Eye ointment.
(Kee J, Hayes E: *Pharmacology: A Nursing
Process Approach,* 1993, p 469. Philadel-
phia, WB Saunders Co.)

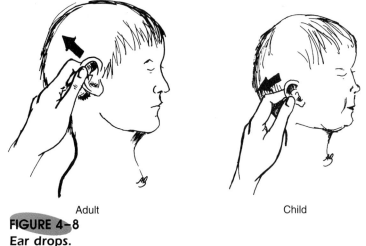

Adult   Child

FIGURE 4-8
Ear drops.
(Kee J, Hayes E: *Pharmacology: A Nursing Process Approach,* 1993, p 471. Philadelphia, WB Saunders Co.)

● Straighten the external ear canal (Fig. 4–8).
   a. *Adult:* Pull the auricle of the ear up and back.
   b. *Child:* Pull the auricle of the ear down and back.
● Instill the prescribed number of drops. Avoid contaminating the dropper.
● Instruct the client to remain in this position for 2 to 5 minutes to prevent the drop from leaking out of the ear.

PHARYNGEAL SPRAY, MOUTHWASH, AND LOZENGE

PURPOSE: Sprays, mouthwashes, and lozenges can be prescribed to reduce throat irritation and for antiseptic and anesthetic effects. These methods are prescribed for a local effect on the throat and *not* for systemic use.

METHODS:

Pharyngeal Spray:

● Instruct the client to sit upright.
● Place a tongue blade over the client's tongue to prevent the tongue from getting numb if an anesthetic is being administered.
● Hold the spray pump nozzle outside the client's mouth and direct the spray to the back of the throat.

Pharyngeal Mouthwash:

● Instruct the client to sit upright.

● Instruct the client to swish the solution around the mouth, but *not* to swallow the solution. The solution is spit into an emesis basin or sink.

Pharyngeal Lozenge:

● Instruct the client to sit upright.

● Instruct the client to place the lozenge in his or her mouth and suck until it is fully dissolved. The lozenge should *not* be chewed or swallowed whole.

TOPICAL PREPARATIONS: LOTION, CREAM, AND OINTMENT

PURPOSE: Topical lotions, creams, and ointments are useful to protect skin areas, prevent skin dryness, treat itching of skin areas, and relieve pain.

METHODS:

Topical Lotion:

● Cleanse skin area with soap and water or other designated solution.

● Shake the lotion container. Use clean or sterile gloves to apply the medicated lotion. Rub the lotion thoroughly into the skin unless otherwise indicated.

Topical Cream and Ointment:

● Cleanse the skin area.

● Use clean or sterile glove(s) and a sterile tongue blade or gauze to apply the cream or ointment to the affected skin area. Use long, smooth strokes. A sterile gauze can be applied to the medicated area after application to prevent soiling clothing.

RECTAL SUPPOSITORY

PURPOSE: Rectal medications are used to relieve vomiting when the client is unable to take oral medication, to relieve pain or anxiety, to promote defecation, and to administer drugs that could be destroyed by digestive enzymes.

METHODS:

● Place the client on his or her left side in the Sims position.

● Use gloves or a finger cot on the index finger.

● Expose the anus by lifting the upper portion of the buttock.

● Lightly lubricate the suppository and insert the narrow (pointed) end of the suppository through the anal sphincter muscle.
● Instruct the client to remain in a supine position for 5 to 10 minutes.

VAGINAL SUPPOSITORY, CREAM, AND OINTMENT

PURPOSE: Vaginal medications are used to treat vaginal infection or inflammation.

METHODS:

● Wear clean gloves.
● Place the client in lithotomy position (knees bent with feet on the table or bed).

Vaginal Suppository:

● Place the suppository at the tip of the applicator.

Vaginal Cream and Ointment:

● Connect the top of the medication tube with the tip of applicatory. Squeeze the tube to fill the applicator.

For All Vaginal Preparations:

● Lubricate the applicator with water-soluble lubricant if necessary.
● Insert applicator downward first and then upward and backward.
● A light pad may be used in the underwear to prevent soiling of clothing. Bedtime is the suggested time for vaginal drug administration.
● Instruct the client to avoid using tampons after insertion of the vaginal medication.

Methods of Calculation

OBJECTIVES

- Determine the amount of drug needed for a specified period of time.

- Select a dosage formula, such as basic formula, ratio and proportion, fraction equation, or dimensional analysis for solving drug dosage problems.

- Convert units of measurement to the same system and unit of measurement prior to calculating drug dosage.

- Calculate the dosage amount of tablets, capsules, and liquid volume (oral or parenteral) needed to administer the prescribed drug.

- Calculate the drug dosage needed according to body weight and body surface area.

Before calculating drug dosage, units of measurement must be converted to one system. If the drug is ordered in milligrams and comes in grains, then grains are converted to milligrams or milligrams are converted to grains.

Four methods for calculating drug dosages are basic formula, ratio and proportion, fractional equation, and dimensional analysis. For drugs that require individualized dosing, body weight and body surface area are used. When body weight and body surface area calculations are used, one of the first three methods for calculation is necessary to determine the amount of drug needed from the container.

At some institutions, the nurse orders enough medication doses for a designated period of time. If the order requires 2 tablets, qid (4 times a day) for 5 days, then the number of tablets needed would be 2 tablets × 4 times a day × 5 days = 40 tablets.

DRUG CALCULATION

The four methods as mentioned for drug calculations are (1) basic formula, (2) ratio and proportion, (3) fractional equation, and (4) dimensional analysis (factor labeling).

Method 1: Basic Formula

The following formula is often used to calculate drug dosages. The basic formula is the most commonly used method, and it is easy to remember.

$$\frac{D}{H} \times V = \text{amount to give}$$

D or desired dose: Drug dose ordered by physician.

H or on-hand dose: Drug dose on label of container (bottle, vial, ampule).

V or vehicle: Form and amount in which the drug comes (tablet, capsule, liquid).

EXAMPLES

PROBLEM 1: Order: cephalexin 1 g, po, bid. Drug available:

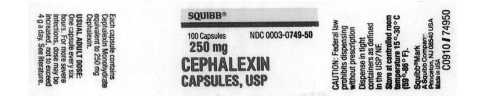

    a. Both the dosage of the drug ordered and the dosage on the bottle are in the metric system; however, the units of measurement are different. Conversion is needed. To convert grams to milligrams, move the decimal point three spaces to the right (see Chap. 1, Metric System).

$$1.0 \text{ g} = 1.000 \text{ mg} = 1000 \text{ mg}$$

b. $\dfrac{D}{H} \times V = \dfrac{\overset{4}{\cancel{1000}}}{\underset{1}{\cancel{250}}} \times 1 \text{ cap} = 4$

Answer: cephalexin 1 g = 4 capsules.

PROBLEM 2: Order: 0.5 g of ampicillin (Principen), po, bid.
Drug available:

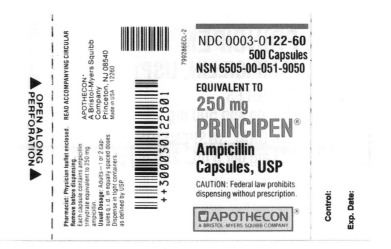

a. The unit of measurement that is ordered and the unit on the bottle are in the same system but in different units; therefore, conversion of units within the same system must be done first. To convert grams to milligrams, move the decimal point three spaces to the right (see Chap. 1, Metric System).

$$0.5 \text{ g} = 0.500 \text{ mg} = 500 \text{ mg}$$

b. $\dfrac{D}{H} \times V = \dfrac{500}{250} \times 1 \text{ capsule} = \dfrac{\overset{2}{\cancel{500}}}{\underset{1}{\cancel{250}}} = 2 \text{ capsules}$

Answer: ampicillin (Principen) 0.5 g = 2 capsules.

PROBLEM 3: Order: phenobarbital gr ii, STAT.
Drug available: phenobarbital 30 mg per tablet.

a. Before calculating drug dosage, convert to one unit of measurement. To convert grains to milligrams, *multiply* the number of grains by 60 (see Chap. 2, Grains and Milligrams).

$$2 \text{ gr} \times 60 = 120 \text{ mg}$$

b. $\dfrac{D}{H} \times V = \dfrac{120}{30} \times 1 = \dfrac{120}{30} = 4 \text{ tablets}$

Answer: phenobarbital gr ⅱ = 4 tablets.

PROBLEM 4: Order: meperidine (Demerol) 35 mg, IM, STAT.
            Drug available:

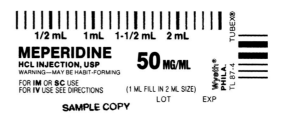

a. Conversion is not needed, because both are of the same unit of measurement.

b. $\dfrac{D}{H} \times V = \dfrac{35}{50} \times 1 \text{ mL} = \dfrac{35}{50} = 0.7 \text{ mL}$

Answer: meperidine (Demerol) 35 mg = 0.7 mL

Method 2: Ratio and Proportion

This is the oldest method used for calculating dosage problems.

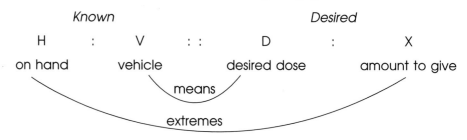

H and **V**: On the left side of the equation are the known quantities, which are dose on hand and vehicle.

D and **X**: On the right side of the equation are the desired dose and the unknown amount to give.

Multiply the means and the extremes. Solve for X.

EXAMPLES

PROBLEM 1: Order: cephalexin 1 g, po, bid.
            Drug available:

Each capsule contains Cephalexin Monohydrate equivalent to 250 mg Cephalexin.

USUAL ADULT DOSE: One capsule every six hours. For more severe infections, dose may be increased, not to exceed 4 g a day. See literature.

SQUIBB®

100 Capsules   NDC 0003-0749-50
250 mg
CEPHALEXIN
CAPSULES, USP

CAUTION: Federal law prohibits dispensing without prescription

Dispense in tight containers as defined in the USP/NF.

Store at controlled room temperature 15°-30°C (59°-86°F).

Squibb®Mark
A Squibb Company
Princeton, NJ 08540 USA
Made in USA

C0910 I 74950

a. To convert grams to milligrams, move the decimal point three spaces to the right (see Chap. 1, Metric System).

$$1.0 \text{ g} = 1.000 \text{ mg} = 1000 \text{ mg}$$

b.

H	:	V	: :	D	:	X
250 mg	:	1 capsule	: :	1000 mg	:	X capsule

$$250 \text{ X} = 1000$$
$$X = 4 \text{ capsules}$$

Answer: cephalexin 1 g = 4 capsules.

Note: With ratio and proportion, the ratio on the left (milligrams to capsules) has the same relation as the ratio on the right (milligrams to capsules); the only difference is values.

PROBLEM 2: Order: aspirin (ASA) gr x, PRN.
Drug available: aspirin 325 mg per tablet.
a. To convert to one system and unit of measurement. To convert grains to milligrams, *multiply* the number of grains by 60 (65) (see Chap. 2, Grains and Milligrams).

$$10 \text{ gr} \times 60 \text{ (65)} = 600 \text{ or } 650 \text{ mg}$$

or

gr	:	mg	: :	gr	:	mg
1	:	60 (65)	: :	10	:	X

$$X = 600 \text{ or } 650 \text{ mg}$$

b.

H	:	V	: :	D	:	X
325 mg	:	1 tablet	: :	600 (650) mg	:	X tablet

$$325 \text{ X} = 600 \text{ (650)}$$
$$X = 1.8 \text{ tablets or 2 tablets}$$
(round off or use 650 instead of 600)

Answer: aspirin gr X = 2 tablets.

PROBLEM 3: Order: amoxicillin 75 mg, po, qid.
Drug available (see page 76):

a. Conversion is not needed because both use the same unit of measurement.

b.

H	:	V	: :	D	:	X
125 mg	:	5 mL	: :	75 mg	:	X mL

$$125 \text{ X} = 375$$
$$X = 3 \text{ mL}$$

Answer: amoxicillin 75 mg = 3 mL.

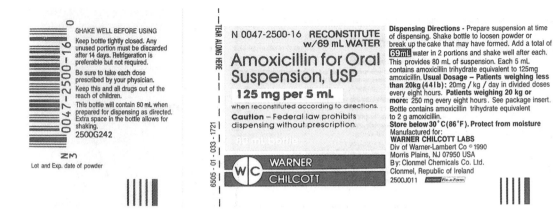

PROBLEM 4: Order: meperidine (Demerol) 60 mg, IM, STAT.
Drug available: Meperidine in a prefilled syringe.

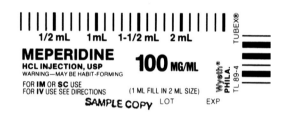

a. Conversion is not needed; the same unit of measurement is used.

b.

H	:	V	: :	D	:	X
100 mg	:	1 mL	: :	60 mg	:	X mL

$$100 X = 60$$
$$X = 0.6 \text{ mL}$$

Answer: meperidine (Demerol) 60 mg = 0.6 mL.

Method 3: Fractional Equation

This method is *similar* to ratio and proportion, except it is written as a fraction.

$$\frac{H}{V} = \frac{D}{X}$$

H: The dosage on hand or on the container.

V: The vehicle or the form in which the drug comes (tablet, capsule, liquid).

D: The desired dosage.

X: The unknown amount to give.

Cross-multiply and solve for **X.**

PROBLEM 1:　Order: cephalexin 1 g, po, bid.
　　　　　　　Drug available:

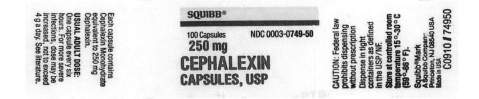

　　a. Convert grams to milligrams. Move the decimal point
　　　　three spaces to the right.

$$1.0 \text{ g} = 1.000 \text{ mg} = 1000 \text{ mg}$$

　　b. $\dfrac{H}{V} = \dfrac{D}{X}$　　　　$\dfrac{250 \text{ mg}}{1 \text{ capsule}} = \dfrac{1000}{X}$

$$250 \text{ X} = 1000$$

$$X = 4$$

Answer: cephalexin 1 g = 4 capsules.

PROBLEM 2:　Order: valproic acid (Depakene) 100 mg, po, tid.
　　　　　　　Drug available: valproic acid (Depakene) 250 mg/5 mL
　　　　　　　suspension.

　　a. No unit conversion is needed.

　　b. $\dfrac{H}{V} = \dfrac{D}{X}$　　　　$\dfrac{250}{5} = \dfrac{100}{X}$

$$250 \text{ X} = 500$$

$$X = 2 \text{ mL}$$

Answer: valproic acid (Depakene) 100 mg = 2 mL.

PROBLEM 3:　Order: atropine gr $^{1}/_{100}$, IM, STAT.
　　　　　　　Drug available:

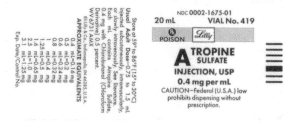

　　a. Two systems are involved: apothecary (grains) and
　　　　metric (milligrams). Because the drug preparation is in

milligrams, convert grains to milligrams (see Table 2–1 or Table 5–1; 0.6 mg = gr $^1/_{100}$).

Also, you could use the ratio method.

$$gr \quad : \quad mg \quad :: \quad gr \quad : \quad mg$$

$$1 \quad : \quad 60 \quad :: \quad ^1/_{100} \quad : \quad X$$

$$X = {}^{60}/_{100}$$

$$X = 0.6 \text{ mg}$$

b. $\dfrac{H}{V} = \dfrac{D}{X}$ $\dfrac{0.4}{1} = \dfrac{0.6}{X}$

$$0.4 X = 0.6$$

$$X = 1.5 \text{ mL}$$

Answer: Atropine gr $^1/_{100}$ = 1.5 mL.

Method 4: *Dimensional Analysis*

The dimensional analysis method (also called factor labeling or the label factor method) calculates dosages using three factors:

1. **Drug label factor:** The form of the drug dose (V) with its equivalence in units (H), e.g., 1 capsule = 250 mg.

2. **Conversion factor (C):** It will help if you memorize the following common conversions:

$$1 \text{ g} = 1000 \text{ mg}$$

$$1 \text{ g} = \quad 15 \text{ gr}$$

$$1 \text{ gr} = \quad 60 \text{ mg}$$

3. **Drug order factor:** The dosage desired (D).

These three factors are set up in an equation that allows you to cancel the units, giving you the correct answer in the correct units for delivery.

$$V = \dfrac{V \text{ (vehicle)} \times \quad C \text{ (H)} \quad \times \text{ D (desired)}}{H \text{ (on hand)} \times \quad C \text{ (D)} \quad \times \quad 1}$$

(drug label)   (conversion factor)   (drug order)

As with other methods for calculation, the three components, D, H, and V, are necessary to solve the drug problem. With dimensional analysis, the conversion factor is built into the equation and is included when the units of measurements of the drug order and drug container differ. If the two are of the same units of measurement, the conversion factor is eliminated from the equation.

EXAMPLES

PROBLEM 1: Order: cephalexin 1 g, po, bid.
                 Drug available:

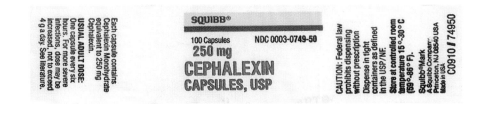

Factors: 250 mg = 1 capsule (from drug label)

1 g/l (from drug order)

Conversion factor: 1 g = 1000 mg

$$cap = \frac{1\ cap \times \overset{4}{\cancel{1000}\ \cancel{mg}} \times 1\ \cancel{g}}{\underset{1}{\cancel{250}\ \cancel{mg}} \times 1\ \cancel{g} \times 1}$$

(drug label) × (conversion factor) × (drug order)

(cancel units and numbers from numerator and denominator)

1 cap × 4 = 4 caps

Answer: cephalexin 1 g = 4 capsules.

PROBLEM 2: Order: quinidine 100 mg, po, bid.

Drug available:

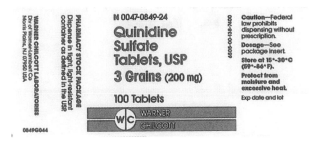

Note: Label is provided for educational purposes; this product has been discontinued by the manufacturer.

Factors: 3 gr = 1 tablet (from drug label)

100 mg/1 (from drug order)

Conversion factor: 1 gr = 60 mg (approximate)

How many tablet(s) would you give?

$$tab = \frac{1\ tab \times 1\ \cancel{gr} \times \overset{5}{\cancel{100}\ \cancel{mg}}}{\underset{3}{3\ \cancel{gr} \times \cancel{60}\ \cancel{mg}} \times 1}$$

$$= \frac{tab \times 5}{3 \times 3} = \frac{5}{9}\ tab = 9\overline{)5.0}^{0.5}\ or\ \frac{1}{2}\ tab$$

Answer: quinidine 100 mg = 0.5 or ½ tablet.

This same problem can be solved by using milligrams, which are also stated on the drug label: The second factor (conversion factor) is *not* needed, because the drug order is in milligrams. Conversion is not necessary, because

$$ tab = \frac{1\ tab \times \overset{1}{\cancel{100}\ \cancel{mg}}}{\underset{2}{\cancel{200}\ \cancel{mg}} \times 1} = 0.5\ or\ \frac{1}{2}\ tablet $$

(drug label) × (drug order)

CALCULATION FOR INDIVIDUALIZED DRUG DOSING

The two methods for individualizing drug dosing are body weight and body surface area (BSA).

Body Weight

Body weight allows the drug dose to be individualized and is often used for children and patients receiving chemotherapy. The first step is to convert pounds to kilograms (if necessary). The second step is to determine the drug dose per body weight by multiplying drug dose × body weight × frequency (day or per day in divided doses). The third step is to choose one of the three methods of drug calculation for the amount of drug to be given.

EXAMPLES

PROBLEM 1 Order: fluorouracil (5-FU), 12 mg/kg/day IV, not to exceed 800 mg/day. The adult weighs 140 pounds.

    a. Convert pounds to kilograms. Divide number of pounds by 2.2.
    Remember: 1 kg = 2.2 lb

$$ 140 \div 2.2 = 64\ kg $$

    b. mg × kg × 1 day =
       12 × 64 × 1   = 768 mg IV per day

Answer: fluorouracil (5-FU), 12 mg/kg/day = 768 mg or 750 to 800 mg.

PROBLEM 2: Give cefaclor (Ceclor), 20 mg/kg/day in three divided doses. The child weighs 20 pounds.

    a. Convert pounds to kilograms.

$$ 20 \div 2.2 = 9\ kg $$

    b. 20 mg × 9 kg × 1 day = 180 mg per day.

$$ 180\ mg \div 3\ divided\ doses = 60\ mg $$

    c. The bottle is labeled 125 mg/5 mL.

BODY SURFACE AREA FOR ADULTS — NOMOGRAM

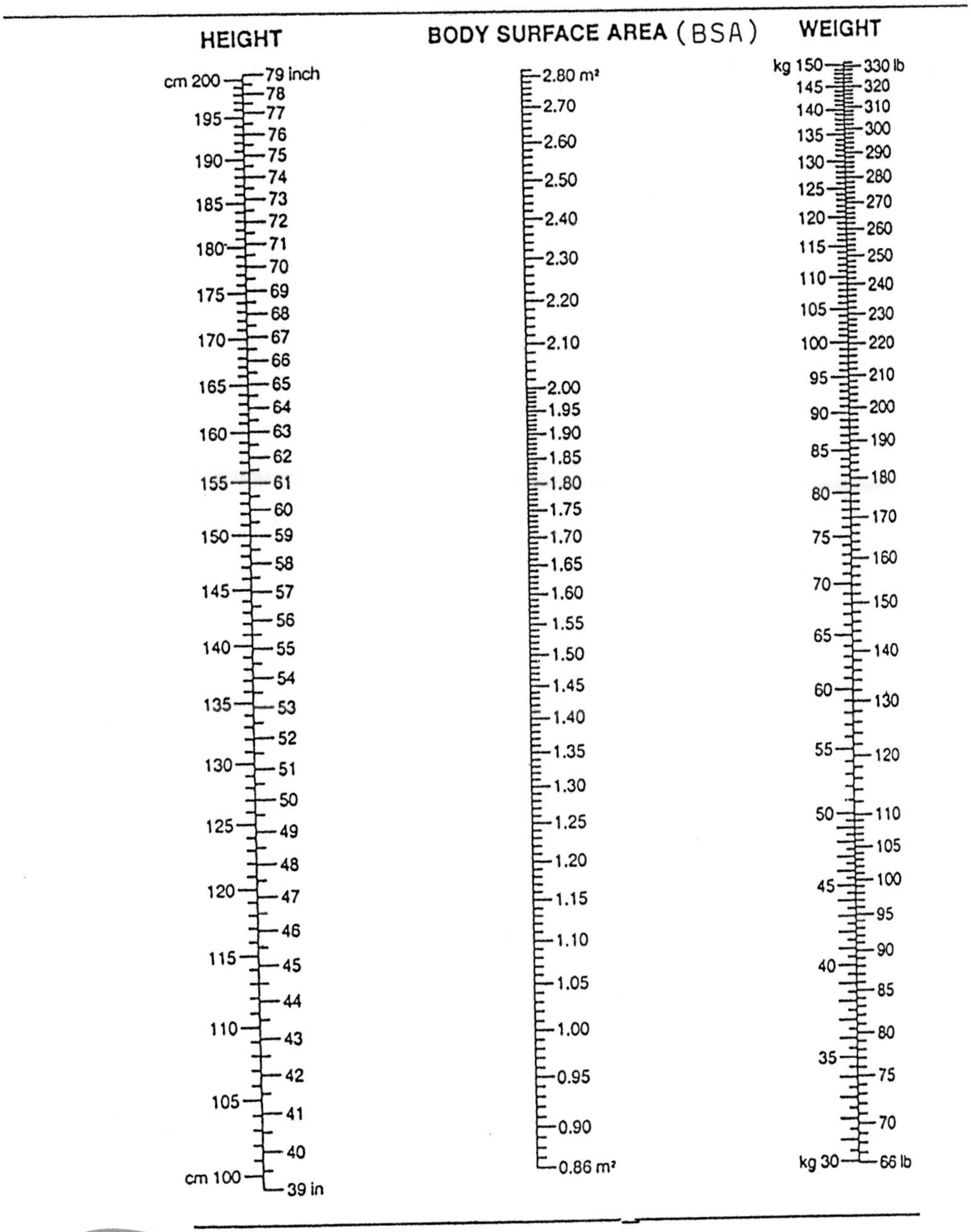

HEIGHT	BODY SURFACE AREA (BSA)	WEIGHT

FIGURE 5-1

Body Surface Area (BSA) Nomogram for Adults

Directions: (1) Find height. (2) Find weight. (3) Draw a straight line connecting the height and weight. Where the line intersects on the BSA column is the body surface area (m²). (From Deglin, J. H., Vallerand, A. H., and Russin, M. M. (1991). *Davis's Drug Guide for Nurses,* 2nd ed. Philadelphia: F. A. Davis, p. 1218. Used with permission from Lentner C. (ed.) (1981). *Geigy Scientific Tables,* 8th ed., Vol. 1. Basel, Switzerland: Ciba-Geigy, pp. 226–227.

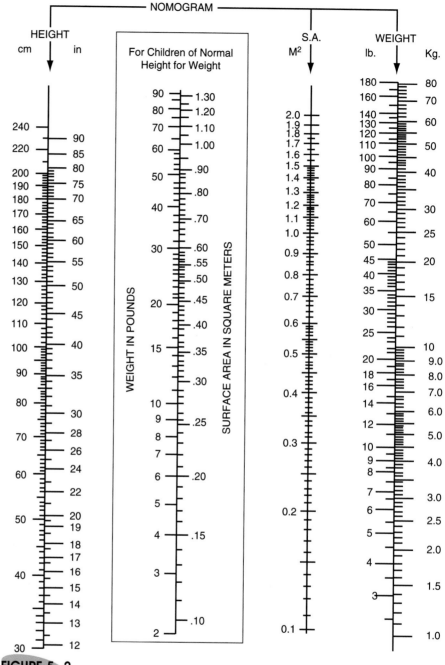

FIGURE 5-2

West Nomogram for Infants and Children

Directions: (1) Find height. (2) Find weight. (3) Draw a straight line connecting the height and weight. Where the line intersects on the SA column is the body surface area (m²). (Modified from data of E. Boyd and C. D. West, in Behrman, R. E. and Vaughan, V. C. (1992). *Nelson Textbook of Pediatrics,* 14th ed. Philadelphia, W. B. Saunders.)

$$\frac{D}{H} \times V = \frac{60}{125} \times 5 \quad \textbf{or} \quad \begin{array}{c} H \; : \; V \; :: \; D \; : \; X \\ 125 \; : \; 5 \; :: \; 60 \; : \; X \end{array} \quad \textbf{or} \quad \frac{125}{5} = \frac{60}{X}$$

$$= \frac{300}{125} = 2.4 \text{ mL} \qquad\qquad \begin{array}{c} 125\,X = 300 \\ X = 2.4 \text{ mL} \end{array} \qquad \begin{array}{c} 125\,X = 300 \\ X = 2.4 \text{ mL} \end{array}$$

Answer: cefaclor (Ceclor) 20 mg/kg/day = 2.4 mL per dose three times per day.

Body Surface Area

BSA is considered to be the most accurate way to calculate drug dosage for infants and children, as well as for patients receiving chemotherapy. The BSA in square meters (m^2) is determined by the person's height and weight and where these intersect on the nomogram scale (Figs. 5–1 and 5–2). To calculate drug dosage by BSA, multiply the drug dose $\times m^2$, e.g., 100 mg $\times 1.6 = 160$ mg/day.

EXAMPLES

PROBLEM 1: Order: cyclophosphamide (Cytoxan) 100 mg/m^2/day, po. Patient weighs 150 pounds and is 5'8" (68 inches) tall.

    a. 68 inches and 150 pounds intersect the nomogram scale at 1.88 m^2 (BSA).

    b. 100 mg $\times$ 1.88 = 188 mg/day of Cytoxan.

Answer: cyclophosphamide (Cytoxan) 100 mg/m^2/day = 188 mg/day.

PROBLEM 2: Order: cytarabine (Cytosine) 200 mg/m^2/day IV $\times$ 5 days for a patient with myelocytic leukemia. The patient is 64 inches tall and weighs 130 pounds.

    a. 64 inches and 130 pounds intersect the nomogram scale at 1.7 m^2 (BSA).

    b. 200 mg $\times$ 1.7 = 340 mg IV daily for 5 days.

Answer: cytarabine (Cytosine) 200 mg/m^2/day = 340 mg/day.

SUMMARY PRACTICE PROBLEMS

Solve the following calculation problems, using method 1, 2, or 3. To convert units within the metric system (grams to milligrams) refer to Chapter 1. To convert apothecary to metric systems and vice versa, refer to Chapter 2 or Table 5–1. For reading drug labels, refer to Chapter 3. Several of the calculation problems have drug labels. Drug dosage and drug form are printed on the drug label.

Extra practice problems are available in the chapters on oral drugs, injectable drugs, and pediatric drug administration.

TABLE 5-1
Metric and Apothecary Conversions*

	METRIC		APOTHECARY
	GRAMS (g)	MILLIGRAMS (mg)	GRAINS (gr)
	1	1000	15
	0.5	500	7½
	0.3	300 (325)	5
	0.1	100	1½
	0.06	60 (64)	1
	0.03	30 (32)	½
	0.015	15 (16)	¼
	0.010	10	⅙
	0.0006	0.6	1/100
	0.0004	0.4	1/150
	0.0003	0.3	1/200

LIQUID (APPROXIMATE)

30 mL (cc) = 1 oz (fl ℥) = 2 tbsp (T) = 6 tsp (t)
15 mL (cc) = ½ oz = 1 T = 3 t
1000 mL (cc) = 1 quart (qt) = 1 liter (L)
500 mL (cc) = 1 pint (pt)
5 mL (cc) = 1 tsp (t)
4 mL (cc) = 1 fl dr (fl ʒ)
1 mL (cc) = 15 minims = 15 drops (gtt)

* Metric and apothecary equivalents frequently used in drug dosage conversions.

1. Order: lorazepam (Ativan) 1 mg, po, tid.
Drug available:

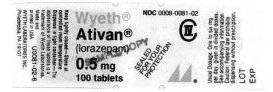

How many tablet(s) would you give? _____

2. Order: sulfisoxazole (Gantrisin) 1 g.
Drug available: sulfisoxazole (Gantrisin) 250 mg per tablet.
How many tablet(s) would you give? _____

3. The physician ordered erythromycin 500 mg, po, q8h, for 7 days.
Drug available: 250 mg tablet.
How many tablets would you order for 7 days? _____
How many tablets would you give every 8 hours? _____

4. Order: ampicillin 100 mg, po, q6h.
Drug available:

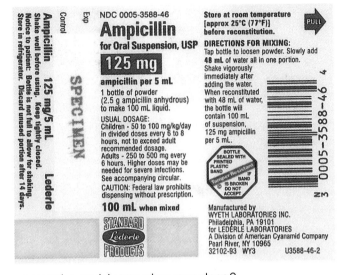

How many mL would you give per dose? _____

5. Order: cephalexin gr 7½ (gr viiss), po, q8h. Drug available:

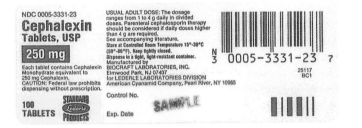

How many tablet(s) would you give per dose? _____

6. Order: methyldopa (Aldomet) 150 mg, po, tid. Drug available:

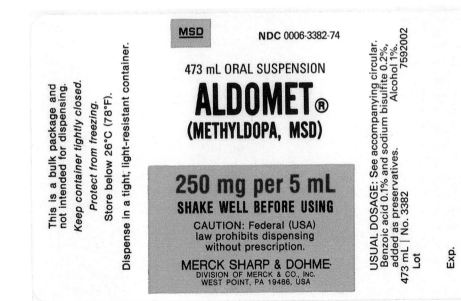

How many mL would you administer? _____

7. Order: dexamethasone (Decadron) 0.5 mg, po, qid.
Drug available:

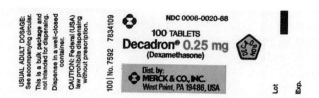

How many tablets would you give per dose? _____
How many milligrams would the patient receive per day?
_____

8. Order: diltiazem (Cardizem) SR 120 mg, po, bid for hypertension.
Drug available:

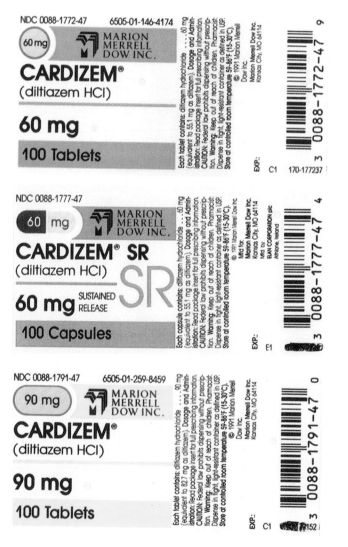

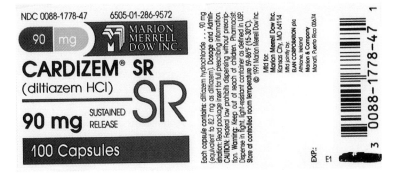

Which drug bottle should be selected? _____
How many tablet(s) should the patient receive per dose?

_____

9. Order: cimetidine (Tagamet) 0.2 g, po, qid.
   Drug available:

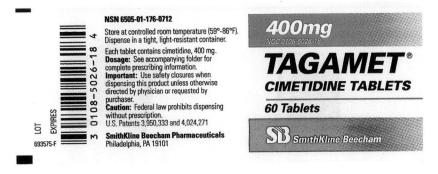

How many tablet(s) would you give per dose? _____

10. Order: codeine gr 1, po, STAT.
    Drug available:

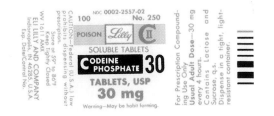

How many tablet(s) should the patient receive? _____

11. Order: methylprednisolone (Medrol) 75 mg, IM.
    Drug available: Medrol 125 mg per 2 mL per ampule.
    How many mL would you give? _____

12. Order: sùlfisoxazole (Gantrisin) 50 mg/kg daily in 4 divided doses
    (q6h). The patient weighs 44 pounds.
    How many milligrams should the patient receive per dose?

_____

13. Order: sulfisoxazole (Gantrisin) 2 g/m² daily in 4 divided doses (q6h). The patient weighs 110 pounds and is 60 inches tall. How many milligrams should the patient receive per dose? _____

14. Order: kanamycin (Kantrex) 15 mg/kg/day in 3 divided doses (q8h), IV. Drug is to be diluted in 100 mg of D₅W. The patient weighs 180 pounds.
Drug available:

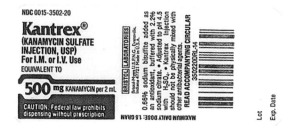

a. How many mg should the patient receive per day? _____

b. How many mg should the patient receive per dose? _____

c. How many mL should the patient receive per dose? _____

15. Order: doxorubicin (Adriamycin) 60 mg/m² IV per month. Patient weighs 120 pounds and is 5'2" (62 inches) tall.
How many milligrams should the patient receive? _____

Dimensional Analysis (Factor Labeling)

16. Order: aminocaproic acid (Amicar) 1.5 g, po, STAT.
Drug available:

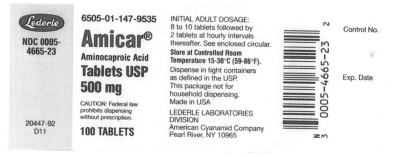

Factors: 500 mg = tablet (drug label)
Conversion factor: 1 g = 1000 mg
How many tablet(s) would you give? _____

17. Order: ampicillin (Principen) 50 mg/kg/day, po, in 4 divided doses (q6h). Patient weighs 88 pounds, or 40 kg (88 ÷ 2.2 = 40 kg). Drug available:

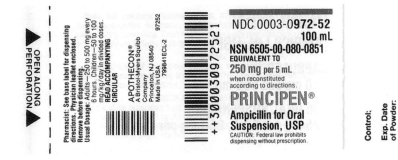

Factors: 250 mg = 5 mL (drug label)
Conversion factor: none (both are in milligrams)
How many milligrams per day should the patient receive?
_____

How many milligrams per dose should the patient receive?
_____

How many milliliters should the patient receive per dose (q6h)?
_____

18. Order: cimetidine (Tagamet) 0.8 g, po, hs.
Drug available:

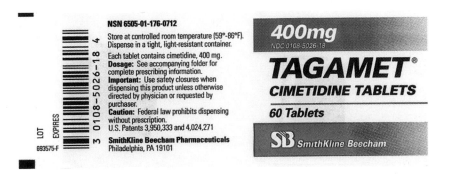

Factors: 400 mg = 1 tablet (drug label)
          0.8 g/1 (drug order)
Conversion factor: 1 g = 1000 mg (units of measurements are not the same; conversion factor is needed)
How many tablet(s) would you give? _____

19. Order: codeine gr i (1), po, STAT.
Drug available:

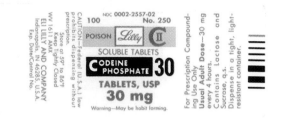

Factors: 30 mg = 1 tablet (drug label)
gr 1/1 (drug order)
Conversion factor: 1 gr = 60 mg
How many tablet(s) would you give? _____

20. Order: amikacin (Amikin) 250 mg, IM, q6h.
Drug available:

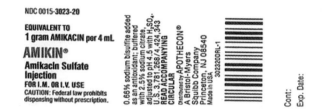

Factors: 1 g = 4 mL (drug label)
250 mg/1 (drug order)
Conversion factor: 1 g = 1000 mg
How many milliliters would you give? _____

ANSWERS:

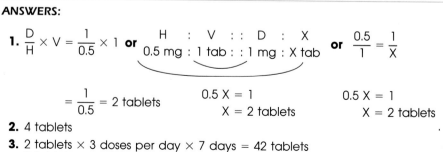

1. $\dfrac{D}{H} \times V = \dfrac{1}{0.5} \times 1$ **or** $\underbrace{\begin{array}{ccccccc} H & : & V & :: & D & : & X \\ 0.5\ mg & : & 1\ tab & :: & 1\ mg & : & X\ tab \end{array}}$ **or** $\dfrac{0.5}{1} = \dfrac{1}{X}$

$= \dfrac{1}{0.5} = 2$ tablets $0.5\ X = 1$ $0.5\ X = 1$
                                                     $X = 2$ tablets $X = 2$ tablets

2. 4 tablets

3. 2 tablets × 3 doses per day × 7 days = 42 tablets
2 tablets every 8 hrs

4. $\dfrac{D}{H} \times V = \dfrac{100}{\underset{25}{\cancel{125}}} \times \dfrac{\cancel{5}^{1}}{1} =$

$$\dfrac{100}{25} = 4 \text{ mL}$$

H : V : : D : X
125 : 5 : : 100 : X

125 X = 500

$$X = \dfrac{500}{125} = 4 \text{ mL}$$

5. Change gr 7½ to grams. Divide the number of grains by 15.

$$7.5 \div 15 = 0.5 \text{ g (see Chap. 2, Grams and Grains)}$$

Change grams to milligrams by moving the decimal three spaces to the right (see Chap. 1, Metric System).

$$0.5 \text{ g} = .500 \text{ mg} = 500 \text{ mg}$$

$\dfrac{D}{H} \times V = \dfrac{500}{250} \times 1$ capsule **or**

$$= \dfrac{500}{250} = 2 \text{ capsules}$$

H : V : : D : X
250 mg : 1 capsule : : 500 mg : X capsule

250 X = 500
X = 2 capsules

6. $\dfrac{D}{H} \times V = \dfrac{150}{\underset{50}{\cancel{250}}} \times \cancel{5}^{1}$ **or**

$$\dfrac{150}{50} = 3 \text{ mL}$$

H : V : : D : X
250 : 5 : : 150 : X

250 X = 750
X = 3 mL

7 a. $\dfrac{D}{H} \times V = \dfrac{0.5}{0.25}$ **or**

$$0.25 \overline{)0.5\,0}^{\,2.} = 2 \text{ tablets}$$

H : V : : D : X
0.25 : 1 tablet : : 0.5 : X tablets

0.25 X = 0.5
X = 2 tablets

  b. 2 mg

8. a. Cardizem SR 60 mg (preferred). Breaking tablets in half does not assure that the patient receives the correct dose.

  b. 2 SR capsules per dose.

9. Change grams to milligrams by moving the decimal three spaces to the right (see Chap. 1, Metric System).

$$0.2 \text{ g} = 0.200 \text{ mg (200 mg)}$$

$\dfrac{D}{H} \times V = \dfrac{200}{400} \times 1$ tablet **or**

$$= \dfrac{200}{400} = ½ \text{ tablet}$$

H : V : : D : X
400 mg : 1 tablet : : 200 mg : X tablet

400 X = 200

$$X = \dfrac{200}{400} = 0.5 \text{ or } ½ \text{ tablet}$$

10. Change grains to milligrams (see Chap. 2 or Table 5–1): 1 gr = 60 mg.

$\dfrac{D}{H} \times V = \dfrac{60}{30} \times 1$ **or**

$$= \dfrac{60}{30} = 2 \text{ tablets}$$

H : V : : D : X
30 mg : 1 tablet : : 60 mg : X tablet

30 X = 60
X = 2 tablets

11. $\dfrac{D}{H} \times V = \dfrac{75}{125} \times 2$ **or** $\quad$ H $\quad$: $\quad$ V $\quad$: : $\quad$ D $\quad$: $\quad$ X $\qquad$ **or** $\quad \dfrac{125}{2} = \dfrac{75}{X}$

$\qquad\qquad\qquad$ 125 $\quad$: $\quad$ 2 $\quad$: : $\quad$ 75 $\quad$: $\quad$ X

$\qquad = \dfrac{150}{125} = 1.2$ mL $\qquad$ 125 X = 150 $\qquad\qquad$ 125 X = 150

$\qquad\qquad\qquad\qquad\qquad\qquad$ X = 1.2 mL $\qquad\qquad\qquad$ X = 1.2 mL

12. Change 44 pounds to kilograms: 44 ÷ 2.2 = 20 kg.

$\qquad$ 50 mg × 20 kg × 1 day = 1000 mg of Gantrisin per day

$\qquad$ 1000 mg ÷ 4 times per day (q6h) = 250 mg q6h

13. 60 inches and 110 pounds intersect the nomogram scale at 1.5 m².

$\qquad$ 2 g × 1.5 m² = 3 g or 3000 mg per day

$\qquad$ 3000 mg ÷ 4 times per day = 750 mg

14. Change 180 pounds to kilograms: 180 ÷ 2.2 = 81.8 kg.

$\quad$ **a.** 15 mg × 82 kg = 1230 mg per day

$\quad$ **b.** 1230 ÷ 3 times a day (q8h) = 410 mg (400 mg, q8h)

$\quad$ **c.** $\dfrac{D}{H} \times V = \dfrac{400}{500} \times 2$ **or** $\quad$ H $\quad$: $\quad$ V $\quad$: : $\quad$ D $\quad$: $\quad$ X

$\qquad\qquad\qquad\qquad\qquad\qquad$ 500 mg $\quad$: $\quad$ 2 mL $\quad$: : $\quad$ 400 mg $\quad$: $\quad$ X mL

$\qquad\qquad = \dfrac{800}{500} = 1.6$ mL $\qquad$ 500 X = 800

$\qquad\qquad\qquad\qquad\qquad\qquad\qquad$ X = 1.6mL

$\quad$ Give kanamycin 1.6 mL.

15. 62 inches and 120 pounds intersect the nomogram scale at 1.6 m².

$\qquad$ 60 mg × 1.6 m² = 96 mg of Adriamycin

16. Tablets = $\dfrac{1 \text{ tablet} \times \overset{2}{\cancel{1000} \text{ m\cancel{g}}} \times 1.5 \text{ \cancel{g}}}{\underset{1}{\cancel{500} \text{ m\cancel{g}}} \times \quad 1 \text{ \cancel{g}} \quad \times \quad 1} = \dfrac{3.0}{1} = 3$ tablets

17. **a.** 50 mg/kg/day

$\qquad$ 50 × 40 = 2000 mg

$\quad$ **b.** 2000 mg ÷ 4 = 500 mg per dose.

$\quad$ **c.** mL = $\dfrac{5 \text{ mL} \times \overset{2}{\cancel{500} \text{ m\cancel{g}}}}{\underset{1}{\cancel{250} \text{ m\cancel{g}}} \times \quad 1} = \dfrac{10}{1} = 10$ mL

18. Tablets = $\dfrac{1 \text{ tablet} \times \overset{10}{\cancel{1000} \text{ m\cancel{g}}} \times 0.8 \text{ \cancel{g}}}{\underset{4}{\cancel{400} \text{ m\cancel{g}}} \times \quad 1 \text{ \cancel{g}} \quad \times \quad 1} = \dfrac{10 \times 0.8}{4} = \dfrac{8}{4} = 2$ tablets

19. Tablets = $\dfrac{1 \text{ tablet} \times \overset{2}{\cancel{60} \text{ m\cancel{g}}} \times 1 \text{ g\cancel{r}}}{\underset{1}{\cancel{30} \text{ m\cancel{g}}} \times \quad 1 \text{ g\cancel{r}} \quad \times \quad 1} = 2$ tablets

20. Milliters = $\dfrac{4 \text{ mL} \times \quad 1 \text{ \cancel{g}} \quad \times \overset{1}{\cancel{250} \text{ m\cancel{g}}}}{1 \text{ \cancel{g}} \quad \times \underset{4}{\cancel{1000} \text{ m\cancel{g}}} \times \quad 1} = \dfrac{4}{4} = 1$ mL

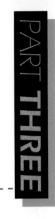

PART THREE

Calculations for Oral, Injectable, and Intravenous Drugs

Oral and Enteral Preparations with Clinical Applications

OBJECTIVES

- State the advantages and disadvantages of administering oral medications.
- Calculate oral dosages from tablets, capsules, and liquids using given formulas.
- Give the rationale for diluting and not diluting oral liquid medications.
- Explain the method for administering sublingual medication.
- Calculate the amount of drug to be given per day in divided doses.
- Determine the amount of tube feeding solution needed for dilution according to the percentage ordered.
- Determine the amount of water needed to dilute liquid medication.

Oral administration of drugs is considered a convenient and economical method to give medications. Oral drugs are available as tablets, capsules, powders, and liquids. Oral medications are referred to as po (per os, or by mouth) drugs and are absorbed by the gastrointestinal tract, mainly from the small intestine.

There are some disadvantages in administering oral medications, such as: (1) variation in absorption rate due to gastric and intestinal pH and food consumption within the gastrointestinal tract; (2) irritation of the gastric mucosa causing nausea, vomiting, or ulceration, e.g., oral potassium chloride; (3) retention or inactivation of the drug in the body because of reduced liver function; (4) destruction of drugs by digestive enzymes; (5) aspiration of drugs into the lungs by seriously ill or confused patients; and (6) discoloration of tooth enamel, e.g., saturated solution of potassium iodide (SSKI). Oral administration is an effective way to give medications in many instances, and at times it is the route of choice.

Body weight and body surface area were discussed in Chapter 5. When solving drug problems that require body weight or body surface area, refer to Chapter 5.

Enteral nutrition and enteral medication are discussed near the end of the chapter. Calculation of percent for enteral feeding solutions and enteral medication are discussed.

TABLETS AND CAPSULES

Most tablets are scored and can be broken in halves and sometimes in quarters. Half of a tablet may be indicated when the drug does not come in a lesser strength.

Capsules are gelatin shells containing powder or time pellets. Time-release capsules should remain intact and not be divided in any way. Many drugs that come in capsules also come in liquid form. When a smaller dose is indicated and is not available in tablet or capsule, the liquid form of the drug is used.

CAUTION:

- A tablet that is NOT scored *should not* be broken.
- Time-release capsules *should not* be crushed and diluted, because the entire medication could be absorbed rapidly.
- Enteric-coated tablets must NOT be crushed, because the medication could irritate the stomach. Enteric-coated tablets are absorbed by the small intestine.
- Tablets or capsules that are irritating to the gastric mucosa should be taken with 6 to 8 ounces of fluid, with meals, or immediately after meals.

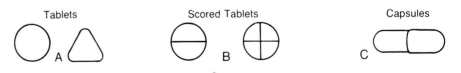

Calculation of Tablets and Capsules

To determine the drug dose, the following steps should be taken:

1. Check the drug order.
2. Determine the drug available (generic name, brand name, and dosage per drug form).
3. Set up method for drug calculation (basic formula, ratio and proportion, fraction equation, or dimensional analysis).
4. Convert to like units of measurement within the same system before solving the problem. Use the unit of measure on the drug container to calculate the drug dose.
5. Solve for the unknown (X).

   Decide which of the methods of calculation you wish to use and then use that same method for calculating all dosages. In the following examples, the basic formula and the ratio and proportion methods are used.

Basic formula	Ratio and proportion

$$\frac{\text{D (desired dose)}}{\text{H (on-hand dose)}} \times V =$$ (vehicle)

$$
\begin{array}{ccccccc}
\text{H} & : & \text{V} & :: & \text{D} & : \text{X} \\
\text{on hand} & & \text{vehicle} & & \text{desired dose} & \text{X}
\end{array}
$$

EXAMPLES

PROBLEM 1: Order: nifedipine (Procardia) 20 mg, tid.
          Drug available: procardia 10 mg per tablet.

Methods: $\dfrac{D}{H} \times V$

$$
\begin{array}{ccccccc}
\text{H} & : & \text{V} & :: & \text{D} & : & \text{X} \\
10\text{ mg} & : & 1\text{ tab} & :: & 20\text{ mg} & : & \text{X tab}
\end{array}
$$

$$\frac{20}{10} \times 1 = 2 \text{ tablets}$$

$$10\,X = 20$$
$$X = 2 \text{ tablets}$$

Answer: Procardia 20 mg = 2 tablets, tid.

PROBLEM 2: Order: ampicillin (Principen) 0.5 g, qid.
          Drug available:

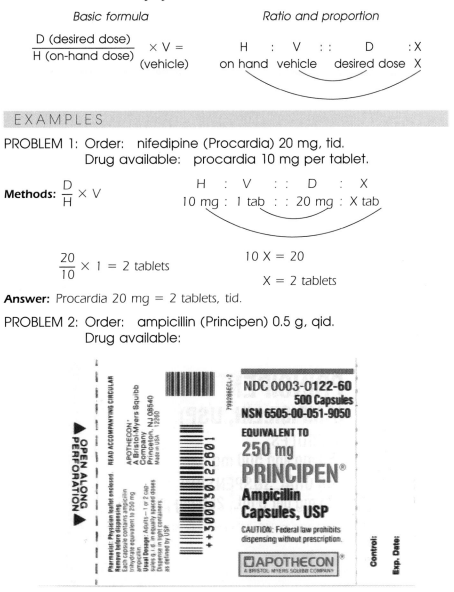

NDC 0003-0122-60
500 Capsules
NSN 6505-00-051-9050

EQUIVALENT TO
250 mg
PRINCIPEN®
Ampicillin
Capsules, USP

CAUTION: Federal law prohibits dispensing without prescription.

☐ APOTHECON®
A BRISTOL-MYERS SQUIBB COMPANY

Control:
Exp. Date:

OPEN ALONG PERFORATION ▲▲

READ ACCOMPANYING CIRCULAR

APOTHECON®
A Bristol-Myers Squibb Company
Princeton, NJ 08540
Made in USA   12260

Pharmacist: Physician leaflet enclosed.
Remove before dispensing.
Each capsule contains ampicillin trihydrate equivalent to 250 mg ampicillin.
Usual Dosage: Adults — 1 or 2 capsules q.i.d. in equally spaced doses. Dispense in tight containers as defined by USP.

Note: Gram (g) and milligram (mg) are both units in the metric system. *Remember:* when changing grams (larger unit) to milligrams (smaller unit), move the decimal point three spaces to the right. Refer to Chapter 1, Table 2–1, or Table 5–1. Because the drug dose on the drug label is in milligrams, conversion should be from grams to milligrams.

Methods: 0.5 g = .500 mg (Method A)

$$\frac{D}{H} \times V = \frac{500}{250} \times 1 \quad \textbf{or} \quad H \ : \ V \ :: \ D \ : \ X$$
$$250 \text{ mg} : 1 \text{ cap} : : 500 \text{ mg} : X \text{ cap}$$

$$= \frac{500}{250} = 2 \text{ capsules} \qquad \begin{array}{c} 250 \text{ X} = 500 \\ X = 2 \text{ capsules} \end{array}$$

Answer: Principen 0.5 g = 2 capsules.

PROBLEM 3: Order: aspirin gr x, po, STAT.
    Drug available: aspirin 325 mg per tablet.

Note: The dose is ordered in the apothecary system, gr x, and the label on the drug bottle is in the metric system (325 mg). Use Table 2–1 or Table 5–1 to convert units.

Methods: 325 mg = gr v (5) and 650 mg = gr x (10)

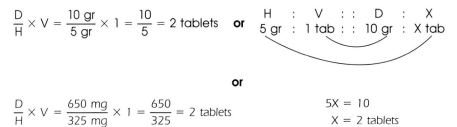

$$\frac{D}{H} \times V = \frac{10 \text{ gr}}{5 \text{ gr}} \times 1 = \frac{10}{5} = 2 \text{ tablets} \quad \textbf{or} \quad \begin{array}{ccccccc} H & : & V & :: & D & : & X \\ 5 \text{ gr} & : & 1 \text{ tab} & : : & 10 \text{ gr} & : & X \text{ tab} \end{array}$$

or

$$\frac{D}{H} \times V = \frac{650 \text{ mg}}{325 \text{ mg}} \times 1 = \frac{650}{325} = 2 \text{ tablets} \qquad \begin{array}{c} 5X = 10 \\ X = 2 \text{ tablets} \end{array}$$

Answer: Aspirin gr x = 2 tablets.

LIQUIDS

Liquid medications come as tinctures, elixirs, suspensions, and syrups. Some liquid medications are irritating to the gastric mucosa and must be well diluted before being given, e.g., KCl (potassium chloride). Usually, liquid cough medicines are not diluted. Medications in tincture form are always diluted.

CAUTION:

- Concentrated liquid medication that can irritate the gastric mucosa should be diluted in *at least* 4 ounces of fluid.
- Liquid medication that can discolor the teeth *should be well diluted and taken through a drinking straw.*

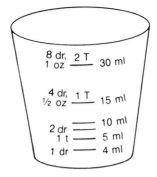

Calculation of Liquid Medications

EXAMPLES

PROBLEM 1: Order: potassium chloride (KCl) 20 mEq, bid.
Drug available: liquid potassium chloride 10 mEq per 5 mL.

Methods: $\dfrac{D}{H} \times V = \dfrac{20}{10} \times 5$ **or** $\begin{array}{ccccccc} H & : & V & :: & D & : & X \\ 10 \text{ mEq} & : & 5 \text{ mL} & :: & 20 \text{ mEq} & : & X \text{ mL} \end{array}$

$= \dfrac{100}{10} = 10 \text{ mL}$ $\begin{array}{c} 10 X = 100 \\ X = 10 \text{ mL} \end{array}$

Answer: Potassium chloride 20 mEq = 10 mL.

PROBLEM 2: Order: tetracycline (Sumycin) 0.25 g, po, tid.
Drug available:

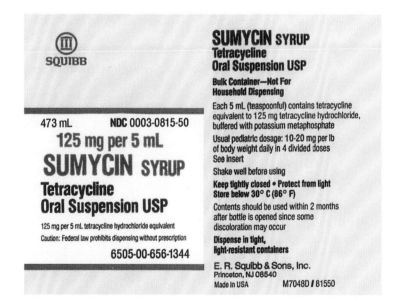

Change grams to milligrams: 0.25 g = 0.250 mg.

Methods: $\dfrac{D}{H} \times V = \dfrac{250}{125} \times 5$ **or**

$$\begin{array}{ccccccc} H & : & V & : : & D & : & X \\ 125\ mg & : & 5\ mL & : : & 250\ mg & : & X\ mL \end{array}$$

$$= \dfrac{1250}{125} = 10\ mL \qquad\qquad 125\ X = 1250$$
$$X = 10\ mL$$

Answer: tetracycline (Sumycin) 0.25 g = 10 mL.

PROBLEM 3: Give SSKI 300 mg, q6h, diluted in water.
　　　　　Available: saturated solution of potassium iodide, 50 mg per drop (gt), drops (gtt).

Methods: $\dfrac{D}{H} \times V = \dfrac{300}{50} \times 1$ **or**

$$\begin{array}{ccccccc} H & : & V & : : & D & : & X \\ 50\ mg & : & 1\ gtt & : : & 300\ mg & : & X\ gtt \end{array}$$

$$= \dfrac{300}{50} = 6\ gtt \qquad\qquad 50\ X = 300$$
$$X = 6\ gtt$$

Answer: SSKI 300 mg = 6 gtt (drops).

SUBLINGUAL TABLETS

　　Few drugs are administered sublingually (tablet placed under the tongue). Sublingual tablets are small and soluble and are quickly absorbed by the numerous capillaries on the underside of the tongue.

CAUTION

　　• *Do not* swallow a sublingual tablet, e.g., nitroglycerin (NTG). If the drug is swallowed, the desired immediate action of the drug is decreased or lost.

　　• Fluids *should not* be taken until the drug has dissolved.

Calculation of Sublingual Medications

EXAMPLES

PROBLEM 1: Order: nitroglycerin (Nitrostat) 0.6 mg, sublingually (SL).
　　　　　Drug available:

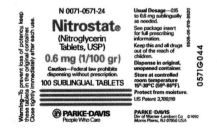

Note: The systems and weights must be the same. See Table 2–1 or Table 5–1. The label has both systems of measurement.

$$0.6\ mg = gr\ \text{\textonequarter{}}... $$

0.6 mg = gr ¹/₁₀₀

Methods:

$$\frac{D}{H} \times V = \frac{0.6}{0.6} \times 1 \quad \textbf{or}$$

$$H \quad : \quad V \quad :: \quad D \quad :$$
$$\frac{1}{100} \text{ gr} : 1 \text{ tab} :: \frac{1}{100} \text{ gr} : X \text{ tab}$$

$$\frac{1}{100} X = \frac{1}{100}$$

$$= \frac{0.6}{0.6} = 1 \text{ SL tablet} \qquad X = \frac{1}{100} \times \frac{100}{1} = 1 \text{ SL tablet}$$

Answer: nitroglycerin (Nitrostat) 0.6 mg = 1 SL tablet.

PROBLEM 2: Order: isosorbide dinitrate (Isordil) 5 mg sublingually.
          Drug available: Isordil 2.5 mg per tablet.

Method: $\frac{D}{H} \times V = \frac{5}{2.5} \times 1$ **or**

$$H \quad : \quad V \quad :: \quad D \quad : \quad X$$
$$2.5 \text{ mg} : 1 \text{ tab} :: 5 \text{ mg} : X \text{ tab}$$
$$2.5 X = 5$$
$$= 2 \text{ SL tablets} \qquad\qquad X = 2 \text{ SL tablets}$$

Answer: Isordil 5 mg = 2 SL tablets.

I. Practice Problems: Oral Medications

For each question, calculate the correct dosage that should be administered.

1. Order: Coumadin 5 mg, po, qd.
   Drug available:

NDC 0056-0176-90

DU PONT PHARMACEUTICALS
COUMADIN® 2½ mg
(crystalline warfarin sodium, U.S.P.)*

HIGHLY POTENT ANTICOAGULANT
WARNING: Serious bleeding results from overdosage. Do not use or dispense before reading directions and warnings in accompanying product information.
USUAL ADULT DOSAGE:
Read accompanying product information.
CAUTION: Federal law prohibits dispensing without prescription.
*Present as crystalline sodium warfarin isopropanol clathrate.
Dispense in a tight, light-resistant container as defined in the U.S.P.
RESEAL CAP TIGHTLY.
PROTECT FROM LIGHT. STORE IN CARTON UNTIL CONTENTS HAVE BEEN USED.
Store at controlled room temperature (59°-86°F, 15°-30°C)
1000 TABLETS

Lot: 3456-T
Exp: 10/5/94

DuPont Pharmaceuticals
E.I. duPont de Nemours & Co.
Wilmington, Delaware 19898
Made and Printed in U.S.A.   7584/CB

a. How many tablet(s) would you give? _____
b. Check the expiration date. Would you give the drug from this bottle? Explain.

2. Order: sulfisoxazole (Gantrisin) 0.5 g.
Drug available: Gantrisin 250 mg per tablet.

3. Order: digoxin (Lanoxin) 0.5 mg.
Drug available:

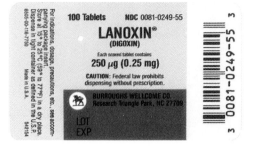

4. Order: codeine gr 1, PRN, q4h.
Drug available:

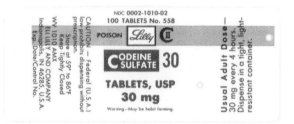

5. Order: potassium chloride 40 mEq, po.
Drug available: potassium chloride 20 mEq/15 mL.

6. Order: (haloperidol) 5 mg, po, bid.
Drug available:

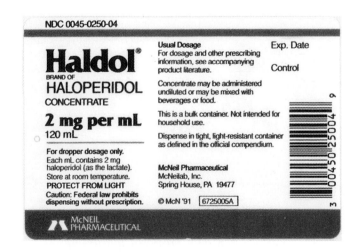

How many mL per dose should the patient receive? _____

7. Order: ProSom (estazolam) 2 mg, po, hs.
Drug available: 1 mg tablet
a. How many tablet(s) should be given? _____
b. What time of day would you administer ProSom? _____

8. Order: ampicillin 500 mg, po, q6h.
Drug available:

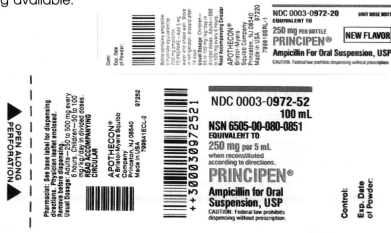

a. How many mL should the patient receive? _____
b. Which drug bottle would you use? _____
Why? _____

9. Order: Artane 3 mg, po, tid.
Drug available:

How many mL should the patient receive? _____

10. Order: HydroDiuril 50 mg, po, qd.
Drug available:

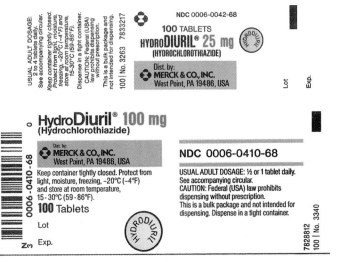

a. Which drug bottle would you use? _____
b. How many tablet(s) would you give, if the tablet(s) are not
scored? _____
Explain. _____

11. Order: Haldol 1 mg, po, tid.
Drug available:

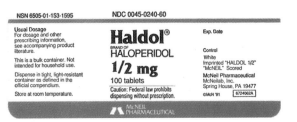

How many tablet(s) should the patient receive? _____

12. Order: cefadroxil (Duricef) 0.4 g, po, q6h.
Drug available:

How many mLs should the patient receive per dose? _____

13. Order: phenobarbital gr s̄s̄.
Drug available: phenobarbital 15 mg per tablet.

14. Order: Penicillin V K (V-Cillin K) 100 mg, po, q6h.
Drug available:

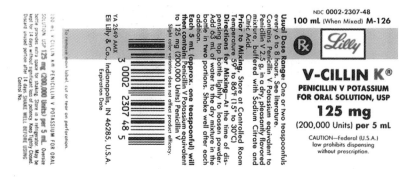

How many mLs should the patient receive per dose? _____

15. Order: meperidine (Demerol) 100 mg, po, q4h, PRN for pain.
Drug available: (unit (individualized) packaged doses)

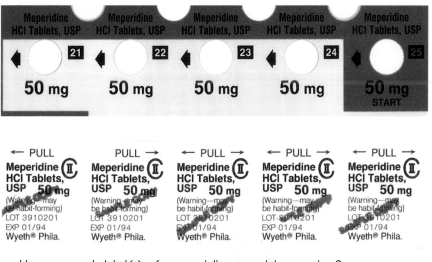

How many tablet(s) of meperidine would you give? _____

16. Order: nitroglycerin gr 1/150, SL, STAT.
Drug available: Nitrostat (nitroglycerin) 0.3 mg, 0.4 mg, 0.6 mg.

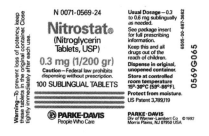

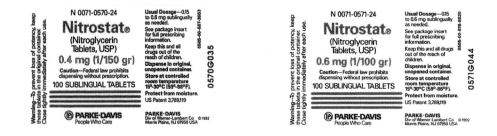

Which Nitrostat SL tablet would you give? (Refer to Table 2–1 or Table 5–1 if needed.) _____

17. Order: Mycostatin 250,000 U oral swish and swallow, qid.
Drug available:

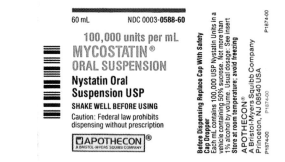

Calculate the correct dosage.

18. Order: diazepam (Valium) 2½ mg.
Drug available: Valium 5 mg scored tablet.
Calculate the correct dosage.

19. Order: Amoxicillin 0.5 g, po, q8h.
Drug available:

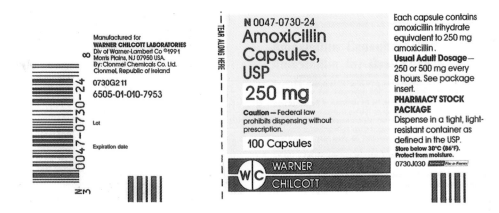

Calculate the correct dosage.

20. Order: allopurinol 450 mg, po, qd.
Drug available: allopurinol 300 mg scored tablet.
Calculate the correct dosage.

21. Order: cefadroxil (Duricef) 1 g, po, as a loading dose; then cefadroxil 0.5 g, po, q12h.
Drug available:

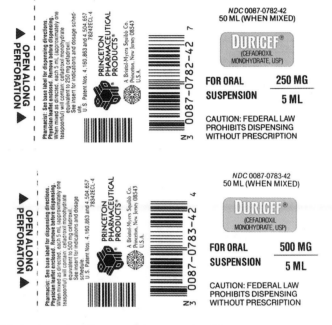

a. Which drug bottle would you select? _____

b. How many milliliters would you give as the loading dose?
_____

c. How many milliliters per 0.5 g? _____

22. Order: lorazepam (Ativan) 0.5 mg, po, q6h.
Drug available: scored tablet.

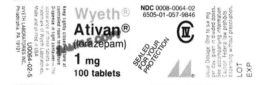

Calculate the correct dosage.

Questions 23-27 relate to body weight and body surface area. Refer to Chapter 5 as necessary.

23. Order: valproic acid (Depakene) 10 mg/kg/day in three divided doses (tid), po. Patient weights 165 pounds. How much Depakene should be administered tid? _____

24. Order: cyclophosphamide (Cytoxan) 4 mg/kg/day, po. Patient weighs 154 pounds. How much Cytoxan would you give per day?
_____

25. Order: mercaptopurine 2.5 mg/kg/day po or 100 mg/m² body surface area po. The patient weighs 132 pounds and is 64 inches tall. The estimated body surface area according to the nomogram is 1.7 m². The amount of drug the patient should receive according to body weight is _____ and according to body surface area is _____ .

26. Order: ethosuximide (Zarontin) 20 mg/kg/day in 2 divided doses (q12h). Patient weighs 110 pounds (100 ÷ 2.2 = 50 kg)
Drug available:

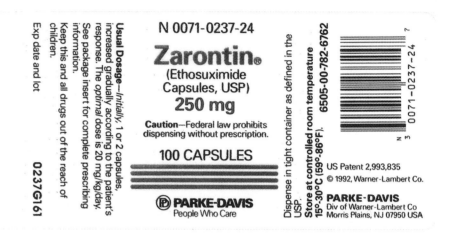

a. How many milligrams should the patient receive per day? ____
b. How many tablet(s) should the patient receive per dose? ____

27. Order: minocycline (Minocin) 4 mg/kg/day in 2 divided doses (q12h). Patient weighs 132 pounds (132 ÷ 2.2 = 60 kg).
Drug available:

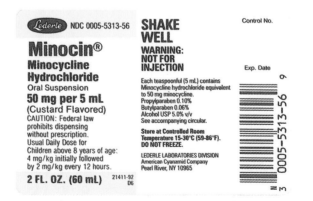

a. How many milligrams should the patient receive per day? ____
b. How many milliliters (mL) should the patient receive per dose?

Questions 28-32 relate to dimensional analysis (factor labeling). Refer to Chapter 5 as necessary.

28. Order: methyldopa (Aldomet) 0.5 g, po, qd.
Drug available: drug label: _____ mg = _____ tablet.

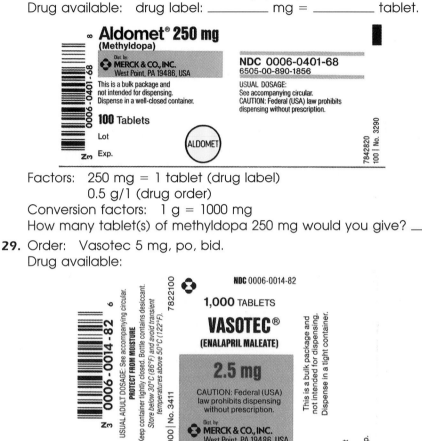

Factors: 250 mg = 1 tablet (drug label)
0.5 g/1 (drug order)
Conversion factors: 1 g = 1000 mg
How many tablet(s) of methyldopa 250 mg would you give? _____

29. Order: Vasotec 5 mg, po, bid.
Drug available:

Factors: 2.5 mg = 1 tablet (drug label); 5 mg/1 (drug order)
Conversion factor: none
How many tablet(s) should the patient receive? _____

30. Order: cephalexin 0.4 g, po, q6h.
Drug available:

Factors: 250 mg/5 mL (drug label); 0.4 g/1 (drug order)
Conversion factor: 1 g = 1000 mg
How many mL would you give? _____

31. Order: acetaminophen (Tylenol) gr x, po.
Drug available:

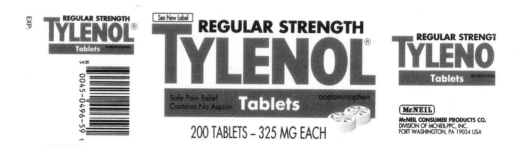

Factors: _____
Conversion factor: _____
How many acetaminophen tablets would you give? _____

32. Order: ampicillin (Principen) 125 mg, po, q6h.
Drug available:

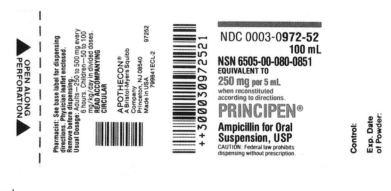

Factors: _____
Conversion factor: _____
How many milliliters of ampicillin (Principen) would you give?

_____

ENTERAL NUTRITION AND DRUG ADMINISTRATION

When the patient is unable to take nourishment by mouth, enteral feeding (tube feeding) is usually preferred over intravenous therapy. Candidates for enteral feedings are patients with neurologic deficits who have difficulty swallowing; debilitated patients; patients with burns and malnutrition disorders; patients having upper gastric obstructions; and patients having radical head and neck surgery. The cost of enteral feedings is much less than intravenous therapy and there is less risk for infection.

Drugs that can be administered orally can be given via enteral tube. The drug must be in liquid form or dissolved into a liquid. The only exceptions are medications in time-release form, enteric-coated form, sublingual form, and bulk-forming laxatives.

Enteral Feedings

Enteral feeding can be administered through a tube inserted into the nose (nasogastric), mouth (orogastric), stomach (gastrostomy), or jejunum (jejunostomy). The nasogastric and orogastric routes are primarily for short-term use and cause nasal and pharyngeal irritation if usage is prolonged. The gastrostomy and jejunostomy routes are for long-term feeding and require a surgical procedure for insertion.

Enteral feedings may be given as a bolus (intermittent) or as a continuous drip feeding over a specified period of time. With bolus feedings, the amount of solution administered is approximately 200 mL or less, and feeding times per day are more frequent. Continuous feedings can be given by gravity flow from a bag or by infusion pump.

There are many types of enteral feeding solutions designed to meet the nutritional needs of patients. Names of common feeding solutions are listed in Table 6–1.

Although enteral feeding solutions are formulated to be given full strength, this strength may not be tolerated. Solutions that are highly concentrated (hyperosmolar or hypertonic) when given in full strength can cause vomiting, cramping, or excessive diarrhea. When gastrointestinal symptoms occur, the enteral solution can be diluted with water. In many situations, patients develop better gastrointestinal tolerance when the strength of the solution is gradually increased. It may take 3 to 5 days for gastrointestinal tolerance to occur. When enteral feedings are less than full strength, they are ordered in percent (%). The nurse must calculate the amount of solution and the amount of water that should be given.

Calculation of Percent for Enteral Feeding Solutions

Percent (%) of a solution indicates its strength. Percent is a portion of 100, e.g., 20% is 20 of 100 parts (20/100). To find percent, the basic formula, ratio and proportion, or a percentage problem can be used.

TABLE 6–1
Common Enteral Formulations

Ensure	Isocal	Nepho
Ensure Plus	Sustacal	Ultracal
Ensure HN	Sustacal HC	Jevity
Osmolite	Vital	Criticare
Osmolite HN	Pulmocare	Promote

D: desired percent

H: on-hand volume (100)

V: desired total volume

X: unknown amount of solution

METHOD A & B Basic formula, and ratio and proportion

$$\frac{D}{H}\left(\frac{\text{desired \%}}{\text{on-hand volume}}\right) \times V \text{ (desired total volume)}$$

or

H : V : : D : X
on-hand : desired : : desired : unknown
volume   total volume   %   amount of
                               solution

or

METHOD C Percentage problem

Desired total volume × desired % (in hundredths) = amount of tube feeding (TF) solution

Following the tube feeding, 30 mL (cc) of water should be given to clear the tubing. The tube is clamped after a bolus feeding.

EXAMPLES

PROBLEM 1: A patient has been receiving intravenous fluids for 5 days. A nasogastric tube was inserted, and 250 mL (cc) of 50% Ensure solution was ordered q4h for 1 day. Calculate how much Ensure and water are needed to make 250 mL (50% solution).

Methods: 50% solution is 50 in 100 parts.

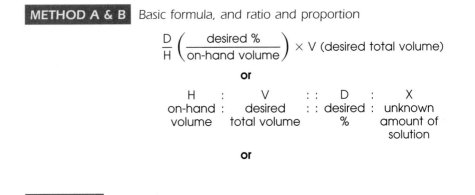

$$\frac{D}{H}\left(\frac{\text{desired \%}}{\text{on-hand volume}}\right) \times \frac{V \text{ (desired}}{\text{total volume)}} \text{ or } \begin{array}{cccc} H : & V & : : D : & X \\ 100 : & 250 \text{ mL} & : : 50 : & X \text{ mL} \end{array}$$

$$\frac{50}{100} \times 250 = \frac{12,500}{100}$$

$$= 125 \text{ mL of Ensure}$$

$$100 X = 12,500$$
$$X = 125 \text{ mL of Ensure}$$

or

250 mL × 0.50 (50%) = 125 mL of TF solution

How much water should be added?

Total amount − amount of TF = amount of water
250 mL   −   125 mL   =   125 mL

Answer: 125 mL of Ensure + 125 mL of water.

PROBLEM 2: Three days later, the patient's tube feeding order is changed. The patient is to receive 250 mL (cc) of 70% Osmolite solution q6h.

How much Osmolite solution and water should be mixed to equal 250 mL?

Methods: 70% solution is 70 in 100 parts.

$$\frac{D}{H} \times V = \frac{70}{100} \times 250 \quad \textbf{or}$$

$$H : V :: D : X$$
$$100 : 250\ mL :: 70 : X\ mL$$

$$= \frac{17,500}{100} = 175\ mL\ of\ Osmolite$$

$$100\ X = 17,500$$
$$X = 175\ mL\ of\ Osmolite$$

or

$$250\ mL \times 0.70\ (70\%) = 175\ mL\ of\ TF\ solution$$

How much water should be added?

Total amount − amount of TF = amount of water
250 mL   −   175 mL   =   75 mL

Answer: 175 mL of Osmolite + 75 mL of water.

PROBLEM 3: One week later, the patient's tube feeding order is changed to 250 mL (cc) of 40% Ensure Plus. How much Ensure Plus and water should be mixed to equal 250 mL?

Methods: 40% solution is 40 in 100 parts.

$$\frac{D}{H} \times V = \frac{40}{100} \times 250 \quad \textbf{or}$$

$$H : V :: D : X$$
$$100 : 250\ mL :: 40 : X\ mL$$

$$= \frac{10,000}{100} = 100\ mL\ of\ Ensure\ Plus$$

$$100\ X = 10,000$$
$$X = 100\ mL\ of\ Ensure\ Plus$$

or

$$250\ mL \times 0.40\ (40\%) = 100\ mL\ of\ TF\ solution$$

How much water should be added?

Total amount − amount of TF = amount of water
250 mL   −   100 mL   =   150 mL

Answer: 100 mL of Ensure Plus + 150 mL of water.

II Practice Problems: Percent of Enteral Solutions

1. Order: 200 mL of 25% Sustacal solution q4h through a nasogastric tube. How much Sustacal solution and water should be mixed to equal 200 mL? _____

2. Order: 300 mL of 75% Pulmocare solution q6h through a nasogastric tube. How much Pulmocare solution and water should be mixed to equal 300 mL? _____

3. Order: 500 mL of 60% Ensure Plus solution q8h through a nasogastric tube. How much Ensure Plus solution and water should be mixed to equal 500 mL? _____

4. Order: 400 mL of 30% Osmolite solution q6h through a nasogastric tube. How much Osmolite solution and water should be mixed to equal 400 mL? _____

Enteral Medications

Oral medications in liquid, tablet, or capsule form can be administered when properly diluted through the feeding tube as a bolus and then flushed from the enteral tube with water. All liquid medication is hyperosmolar (>1000 mOsm/kg) when compared with the osmolality of the secretions of the gastrointestinal tract (130 to 350 mOsm/kg). Although the hyperosmolality of liquid medication was once thought to be well tolerated by the gastrointestinal tract, research indicates that cramping, distention, vomiting, and diarrhea can be caused by the administration of undiluted hypertonic liquid medications and electrolyte solutions. Liquid medication should be diluted with water to reduce osmolality to 500 mOsm/kg to decrease gastrointestinal intolerance.

Table 6–2 lists the osmolalities of various commercial drug solutions and suspensions.

Calculation of Dilution for Enteral Medications

To determine the amount of water needed to dilute a liquid medication, the following information must be obtained:

1. Calculate the drug order to find the volume of the drug.
2. Find the osmolality of the drug (check drug literature or pharmacist).
3. Use 500 mOsm as a constant for the desired osmolality.

METHOD **Step 1** Calculate the volume of drug

$$\frac{D}{H} \times V \quad \textbf{or} \quad H \;:\; V \;::\; D \;:\; X$$

Step 2 Find osmolality of drug

$$\frac{\text{known mOsm}}{\text{desired mOsm}} \times \text{volume of drug} = \text{total volume of liquid}$$

Step 3 Water for dilution

total volume of liquid − volume of drug = volume of water
for dilution

EXAMPLES

PROBLEM 1: Order: acetaminophen 650 mg, q6h, PRN for pain.
         Drug available: acetaminophen elixir 65 mg/mL.
                  Average mOsm/kg = 5400.

TABLE 6-2
Osmolalities of Various Commercial Drug Solutions and Suspensions

PRODUCT	MANUFACTURER	AVERAGE OSMOLALITY (m/Osm/kg)
Acetaminophen elixir, 65 mg/mL	Roxane	5400
Acetaminophen with codeine elixir	Wyeth	4700
Amoxicillin suspension, 50 mg/mL	Squibb	2250
Ampicillin suspension, 50 mg/mL	Squibb	2250
Cascara aromatic fluid extract	Roxane	1000
Cephalexin suspension, 50 mg/mL	Dista	1950
Cimetidine solution, 60 mg/mL	SmithKline French	5500
Co-trimoxazole suspension	Burroughs	2200
Dexamethasone solution, 1 mg/mL	Roxane	3100
Dextromethorphan HBr syrup, 2 mg/mL	Parke-Davis	5950
Digoxin elixir, 50 μg/mL	Burroughs	1350
Diphenhydramine HCl elixir, 2.5 mg/mL	Roxane	850
Diphenoxylate/atropine suspension	Roxane	8800
Docusate sodium syrup, 3.3 mg/mL	Roxane	3900
Erythromycin E.S. suspension, 40 mg/mL	Abbott	1750
Ferrous sulfate liquid, 60 mg/mL	Roxane	4700
Furosemide solution, 10 mg/mL	Hoescht-Roussel	2050
Haloperidol concentrate, 2 mg/mL	McNeil	500
Hydroxyzine HCl syrup, 2 mg/mL	Roerig	4450
Kaolin-pectin suspension	Roxane	900
Lactulose syrup, 0.67 g/mL	Roerig	3600
Lithium citrate syrup, 1.6 mEq/mL	Roxane	6850
Magnesium citrate solution	Medalist	1000
Metoclopramide HCl syrup, 1 mg/mL	Robins	8350
Milk of magnesia suspension	Pharmac. Assoc.	1250
Multivitamin liquid	Upjohn	5700
Nystatin suspension, 100,000 U/mL	Squibb	3300
Paregoric tincture	Roxane	1350
Phenytoin sodium susp., 25 mg/mL	Parke-Davis	1500
Potassium chloride liquid, 10%	Roxane	3550
Potassium iodide sat sol (SSKI), 1 g/mL	Upsher-Smith	10950
Prochlorperazine syrup, 1 mg/mL	SmithKline French	3250
Promethazine HCl syrup, 1.25 mg/mL	Wyeth	3500
Sodium phosphate liquid, 0.5 g/mL	Fleet	7250
Theophyline solution, 5.33 mg/mL	Berlex	800
Thioridazine suspension, 20 mg/mL	Sandoz	2050

(Source: Estoup, Michael (1994). Approaches and limitations of medication delivery in patients with enteral feeding tubes. *Critical Care Nurse*, Vol 14(1), Table 2, p. 70. Reprinted with permission of *Critical Care Nurse*, February, 1994.)

Step 1 Calculate the volume of drug

$$\frac{D}{H} \times V = \frac{650}{65} \times 1 \quad \textbf{or} \quad \begin{array}{ccccccc} H & : & V & :: & D & : & X \\ 65 \text{ mg} & : & 1 \text{ mL} & :: & 650 \text{ mg} & : & X \text{ mL} \end{array}$$

$$= 10 \text{ mL} \qquad\qquad 65 \, X = 650$$
$$X = 10 \text{ mL}$$

Step 2 Find osmolality of drug

$$\frac{\text{known mOsm (5400)}}{\text{desired mOsm (500)}} \times \text{volume of drug (10)} = \frac{5400}{500} \times 10 = 108 \text{ mL}$$

Step 3 Water for dilution

total volume of drug (108 mL) − volume of drug (10 mL)

= 98 mL volume of water for dilution

PROBLEM 2: Order: Colace 50 mg bid.
Drug available: docusate sodium 3.3 mg/mL.
Average mOsm/kg = 3900.

Step 1 Calculate the volume of drug

$$\frac{D}{H} \times V = \frac{50}{3.3} \times 1 \quad \textbf{or} \qquad \begin{array}{ccccc} H & : & V & :: & D & : X \\ 3.3\ mg & : & 1\ mL & :: & 50\ mg & : X \end{array}$$

$$= 15.1\ mL \qquad\qquad\qquad 3.3\ X = 50$$
$$X = 15.1\ or\ 15\ mL$$

Step 2 Find osmolality of drug

$$\frac{known\ mOsm\ (3900)}{desired\ mOsm\ (500)} \times volume\ of\ drug\ (15\ mL) = \frac{3900}{500} \times 15 = 117\ mL$$

Step 3 Water for dilution

total volume of drug (117 mL) − volume of drug (15 mL)

= 102 mL volume of water for dilution

III Practice Problems: Enteral Medications

Calculate the amount of water needed to reduce the osmolality to 500 mOsm for the following medications:

1. Order: amoxicillin suspension 250 mg by tube, qid.
   Drug available: amoxicillin suspension 50 mg/mL.
2. Order: metoclopramide HCl syrup 10 mg, q ac and hs per tube.
   Drug available: metoclopramide 1 mg/mL.
3. Order: KCl oral solution 40 mEq, qd by tube.
   Drug available: KCl 10% oral solution, 20 mEq/15 mL
4. Order: thioridazine suspension 50 mg, tid by tube.
   Drug available: thioridazine suspension 20 mg/mL.

ANSWERS

I. Practice Problems: Oral Medications

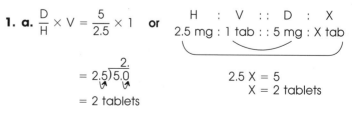

1. a. $\dfrac{D}{H} \times V = \dfrac{5}{2.5} \times 1 \quad \textbf{or} \qquad \begin{array}{ccccc} H & : & V & :: & D & : & X \\ 2.5\ mg & : & 1\ tab & :: & 5\ mg & : & X\ tab \end{array}$

$$= 2.5\overline{)5.0}^{\,2.}$$
$$= 2\ tablets$$

$$2.5\ X = 5$$
$$X = 2\ tablets$$

b. No. Expiration date has expired.

2. 0.5 g = 500 mg (Method A) or see Table 2–1 or Table 5–1.

$$\frac{D}{H} \times V = \frac{500}{250} \times 1 \quad \textbf{or} \quad \begin{array}{c} H \quad : \quad V \quad :: \quad D \quad : \quad X \\ 250\ mg : 1\ tab : : 500\ mg : X\ tab \end{array}$$

$$= \frac{500}{250} = 2\ tablets \qquad \begin{array}{c} 250\ X = 500 \\ X = 2\ tablets \end{array}$$

3. 2 tablets

4. Change grains to milligrams (milligram value is on the drug label). Refer to Chapter 2, Table 2–1, or Table 5–1: 1 gr = 60 mg.

$$\frac{D}{H} \times V = \frac{60}{30} \times 1 \quad \textbf{or} \quad \begin{array}{c} H \quad : \quad V \quad :: \quad D \quad : \quad X \\ 30\ mg : 1\ tab : : 60\ mg : X\ tab \end{array}$$

$$= 2\ tablets \qquad \begin{array}{c} 30\ X = 60 \\ X = 2\ tablets \end{array}$$

5. 30 mL

6. $\dfrac{D}{H} \times V = \dfrac{5}{2} \times 1\ mL \quad \textbf{or} \quad \begin{array}{c} H : V : : D : X \\ 2 : 1 : : 5 : X \end{array}$

$$= 2.5\ mL\ of\ Haldol \quad 2\ X = 5$$
$$X = \frac{5}{2} = 2.5\ mL$$

7. a. 2 tablets of ProSom
   b. hs : hour of sleep or at bedtime.

8. a. 10 mL per dose of ampicillin.
   b. Principen 100 mL bottle. The 500 mg of ampicillin can be poured from this bottle. The 250 mg per bottle is intended for 1 dose of 250 mg. Two 250-mg bottles would be needed for 500 mg; this would be expensive.

9. $\dfrac{D}{H} \times V = \dfrac{3}{2} \times 5\ mL = \dfrac{15}{2} \quad \textbf{or} \quad \begin{array}{c} H : V : : D : X \\ 2 : 5 : : 3 : X \end{array}$

$$= 7.5\ mL\ of\ Artane \qquad 2\ X = 15$$
$$X = 7.5\ mL\ of\ Artane$$

10. a. The HydroDiuril 25 mg tablet bottle is preferred. A half tablet from the HydroDiuril 100 mg tablet bottle can be used; however, breaking or cutting the 100 mg tablet can result in an inaccurate dose.
   b. From the HydroDiuril 25 mg bottle, give 2 tablets. From the Hydro-Diuril 100 mg bottle, give ½ tablet (if the tablet is scored).

11. ½ mg = 0.5 mg.
   Give 2 tablets of Haldol.

12. Change grams to milligrams by moving the decimal point three spaces to the right: 0.400 g = 400 mg. Also see Table 2–1 or Table 5–1.

$$\frac{D}{H} \times V = \frac{400}{250} \times 5\ mL \quad \textbf{or} \quad \begin{array}{c} H \quad : \quad V \quad :: \quad D \quad : \quad X \\ 250\ mg : 5\ mL : : 400\ mg : X\ mL \end{array}$$

$$= \frac{2000}{250} = 8\ mL \qquad \begin{array}{c} 250\ X = 2000 \\ X = 8\ mL \end{array}$$

13. Use the metric system. According to Table 2–1 or Table 5–1, gr $\overline{ss}$ = 30 mg. Give 2 tablets.

14. $\dfrac{D}{H} \times V = \dfrac{100}{125} \times 5 \text{ mL}$ **or** $\begin{array}{ccccc} H & : & V & :: & D & : X \\ 125 \text{ mg} & : & 5 \text{ mL} & :: & 100 \text{ mg} & : X \end{array}$

$\qquad\qquad = \dfrac{500}{125} = 4 \text{ mL}$ $\qquad\qquad \begin{array}{c} 125 \, X = 500 \\ X = 4 \text{ mL} \end{array}$

15. Give 2 tablets of meperidine.

16. Nitrostat 0.4 mg

17. 2½ mL

18. ½ tablet

19. 2 tablets

20. 1½ tablets

21. a. For loading dose and maintenance doses, the 500 mg/5 mL is preferred, but either bottle could be used.
   b. Loading dose: change grams to milligrams.

$$1.000 \text{ g} = 1000 \text{ mg}$$

Using the 250 mg/5 mL bottle

$\dfrac{D}{H} \times V = \dfrac{1000}{\underset{50}{\cancel{250}}} \times \cancel{5}^{\,1} \text{ mL}$ **or** $\begin{array}{ccccc} H & : & V & :: & D & : X \\ 250 \text{ mg} & : & 5 \text{ mL} & :: & 1000 \text{ mg} & : X \text{ mL} \end{array}$

$\qquad\qquad = \dfrac{1000}{50} = 20 \text{ mL}$ $\qquad\qquad \begin{array}{c} 250 \, X = 5000 \\ X = 20 \text{ mL} \end{array}$

Using the 500 mg/5 mL bottle, give 10 mL per dose of Duricef.
   c. Maintenance doses per dose, change grams to milligrams

$$0.500 \text{ g} = 500 \text{ mg}$$

Using the 250 mg/5 mL bottle

$\dfrac{D}{H} \times V = \dfrac{500}{250} \times 5 \text{ mL}$ **or** $\begin{array}{ccccc} H & : & V & :: & D & : X \\ 250 \text{ mg} & : & 5 \text{ mL} & :: & 500 \text{ mg} & : X \end{array}$

$\qquad\qquad = 10 \text{ mL}$ $\qquad\qquad \begin{array}{c} 250 \, X = 2500 \\ X = 10 \text{ mL} \end{array}$

Using the 500 mg/5 mL; give 5 mL per dose of Duricef.

22. ½ tablet

23. 165 lb = 75 kg (change pounds to kilograms by dividing by 2.2 into 165 pounds, or 165 ÷ 2.2)

10 mg × 75 = 750 mg
750 ÷ 3 = 250 mg, tid

24. 154 lb = 70 kg
4 mg × 70 = 280 mg/day

25. 132 lb = 60 kg
2.5 mg × 60 = 150 mg **or** 100 × 1.7 = 170 mg

26. a. 20 mg/50 kg/day = 20 × 50 = 1000 mg per day
   b. 2 tablets of Zarontin per dose (500 mg per dose)

27. a. 4 mg/60 kg/day = 4 × 60 = 240 mg per day **or** 120 mg, q12h

b. $\dfrac{D}{H} \times V = \dfrac{120}{\underset{10}{\cancel{50}}} \times \underset{1}{\cancel{5}}\ mL =$

$= \dfrac{120}{10} = 12\ mL$

H : V : : D : X

50 : 5 : : 120 : X

50 X = 600

$X = \dfrac{600}{50} = 12\ mL$

Give 12 mL per dose of minocycline.

28. Drug label: 250 mg = 1 tablet.

$tablets = \dfrac{1\ tab \quad \times \overset{4}{\cancel{1000}}\ \cancel{mg} \times 0.5\ \cancel{g}}{\underset{1}{\cancel{250}}\ \cancel{mg} \times \quad 1\ \cancel{g} \quad \times \quad 1} = 0.5 \times 4 = 2\ tablets$

29. $tablets = \dfrac{1 \quad \times \overset{2}{\cancel{5.0}}\ \cancel{mg}}{\underset{1}{\cancel{2.5}}\ \cancel{mg} \times \quad 1} = 2\ tablets\ of\ Vasotec$

30. $mL = \dfrac{5\ mL \times \overset{4}{\cancel{1000}}\ \cancel{mg} \times 0.4\ \cancel{g}}{\underset{1}{\cancel{250}}\ \cancel{mg} \times \quad 1 \quad \cancel{g} \quad \times \quad 1} = 8\ mL$

Give 8 mL per dose of cephalexin.

31. Factors: 325 mg = 1 tablet; gr × (10)/1
Conversion factor: 1 gr = 60 mg

$tablets = \dfrac{1\ tab \quad \times \overset{12}{\cancel{60}}\ \cancel{mg} \times \overset{2}{\cancel{10}}\ \cancel{gr}}{\underset{\underset{13}{\cancel{65}}}{\cancel{325}}\ \cancel{mg} \times \quad 1\ \cancel{gr} \quad \times \quad 1} = \dfrac{24}{13} = 1.84\ or\ 2\ tablets$

60 (64) mg = 1 gr (approximate weights). Round off to the nearest whole number.

32. Factors: 250 mg = 5 mL; 125 mg/1
Conversion factor: *none*

$mL = \dfrac{5\ mL \quad \times \overset{1}{\cancel{125}}\ \cancel{mg}}{\underset{2}{\cancel{250}}\ \cancel{mg} \times \quad 1} = \dfrac{5}{2} = 2\frac{1}{2}\ or\ 2.5\ mL$

II. Percent of Enteral Solutions

1. $\dfrac{D}{H} \times V = \dfrac{25}{100} \times 200$ **or** 100 : 200 : : 25 : X

$= \dfrac{200}{4} = 50\ mL\ of$ ⠀⠀ 100 X = 5000
Sustacal ⠀⠀ X = 50 mL of Sustacal

or

200 mL × 0.25 (25%) = 50 mL of Sustacal

Total amount − amount of TF = amount of water
⠀⠀200 mL ⠀⠀ − ⠀⠀ 50 mL ⠀ = ⠀⠀ 150 mL

50 mL of Sustacal + 150 mL of water

2. 225 mL of Pulmocare + 75 mL of water

3. $\dfrac{D}{H} \times V = \dfrac{60}{100} \times 500$ **or** $100 : 500 : : 60 : X$

$= \dfrac{30,000}{100} = 300$ mL of Ensure Plus

$100\,X = 30,000$
$X = 300$ mL of Ensure Plus

or

500 mL $\times 0.60\ (60\%) = 300$ mL of Ensure Plus

Total amount $-$ amount of TF $=$ amount of water
500 mL $\quad - \quad 300$ mL $\quad = \quad 200$ mL

300 mL of Ensure Plus $+ 200$ mL of water

4. 120 mL of Osmolite + 280 mL of water

III. Enteral Medications

1. *Step 1* $\dfrac{D}{H} \times V = \dfrac{\overset{5}{\cancel{250}}}{\underset{1}{\cancel{50}}} \times 1$ **or** $\begin{array}{l} H : V :: D : X \\ 50 : 1 :: 250 : X \end{array}$

$= 5$ mL

$50\,X = 250$
$X = 5$ mL

Step 2 $\dfrac{\text{known mOsm } (2250)}{\text{desired mOsm } (500)} \times$ volume of drug (5)

$= \dfrac{2250}{500} \times 5$ mL $= 22.5$ mL

Step 3 Total volume of liquid $= (22.5) -$ volume of drug $(5) = 17.5$ mL
Total: 22.5 mL to be administered

2. *Step 1* $\dfrac{D}{H} \times V = \dfrac{10}{1} \times 1 = 10$ **or** $\begin{array}{l} H : V :: D : X \\ 1\text{ mg} : 1\text{ mL} :: 10\text{ mg} : X \end{array}$

$X = 10$ mL

Step 2 $\dfrac{\text{known mOsm } (8350)}{\text{desired mOsm } (500)} \times$ volume of drug (10)

$= \dfrac{8350}{500} \times 10 = 167$ mL

Step 3 total volume of liquid (167 mL) $-$ volume of drug
(10 mL) $= 157$ mL

3. *Step 1* $\dfrac{D}{H} \times V = \dfrac{\overset{2}{\cancel{40}}}{\underset{1}{\cancel{20}}} \times 15 = 30$ mL **or** $\begin{array}{l} H : V :: D : X \\ 20\text{ mEq} : 15\text{ mL} :: 40\text{ mEq} : X \end{array}$

$20\,X = 600$
$X = 30$ mL

Step 2 $\dfrac{\text{known mOsm } (3550)}{\text{desired mOsm } (500)} \times$ volume of drug (30)

$= \dfrac{3550}{500} \times 30 = 213$ mL

Step 3 total volume of liquid (213) $-$ volume of drug (30) $= 183$ mL

4. *Step 1* $\dfrac{D}{H} \times V = \dfrac{\overset{50}{\cancel{50}}}{\underset{2}{\cancel{20}}} \times 1 = 2.5 \text{ mL}$ **or** $\begin{array}{ccccc} H & : & V & :: & D & : X \\ 20 \text{ mg} & : & 1 \text{ mL} & :: & 50 \text{ mg} & : X \end{array}$

$$20\,X = 50$$
$$X = 2.5 \text{ mL}$$

Step 2 $\dfrac{\text{known mOsm (2050)}}{\text{desired mOsm (500)}} \times \text{volume of drug (2.5)} = 10.25 \text{ mL}$

Step 3 total volume of liquid (10.25 mL) − volume of drug (2.5 mL)
= 7.75 mL

Injectable Preparations with Clinical Applications

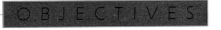

OBJECTIVES

- Select the correct syringe and needle for a prescribed injectable drug.
- Calculate dosage of drugs for subcutaneous and intramuscular routes from solutions in vials and ampules.
- Explain the procedure for preparing and calculating medications in powder form for injectable use.
- Determine prescribed insulin dosage in units using an insulin syringe.
- Explain the methods for mixing two insulin solutions in one insulin syringe and for mixing two injectable drugs in one syringe.
- State the various sites for intramuscular injections.
- Explain how to administer intradermal, subcutaneous, and intramuscular injections.
- Calculate the rate of direct IV injection.

Medications administered by injection can be given intradermally (under the skin), subcutaneously (SC, into fatty tissue), intramuscularly (IM, into the muscle), and intravenously (IV, into the vein). Intravenous injectables are discussed in Chapter 8. Injectable drugs are ordered in grams, milligrams, micrograms, grains, or units. The preparations of injectable drugs may be packaged in a solvent (diluent or solution) or in a powdered form.

This chapter is divided into six sections: (1) injectable preparations, such as vials, ampules, syringes, needles, and prefilled cartridges; (2) intradermal injections; (3) subcutaneous injections, including heparin; (4) insulin injections; (5) intramuscular injections from prepared liquid and reconstituted powder in vials and ampules, and the mixing of drugs in a syringe; and (6) direct IV injection. Examples and practice problems follow each section, and the answers to the practice problems are located at the end of the chapter.

INJECTABLE PREPARATIONS

Vials and Ampules

Drugs are packaged in vials (sealed rubber-top containers) for single and multiple doses and in ampules (sealed glass containers) for a single dose. Multiple-dose vials can be used more than once because of their self-sealing rubber top; however, ampules are used only once after the glass-necked container is opened. The drug is in either liquid or powder form in vials and ampules. When drugs in solution deteriorate rapidly, they are packaged in dry form and solvent (diluent) is added prior to administration. If the drug is in powdered form, mixing instructions and dose equivalents such as milligrams (mg) per milliliter (mL) are usually given; if not, check the drug circular. After the dry form of the drug is reconstituted with sterile water, bacteriostatic water, or saline, the drug is used immediately or must be refrigerated. Usually, the reconstituted drug in the vial is used within 48 hours to 1 week; check the drug circular. Illustrations of a vial and an ampule are displayed in Figure 7–1.

The route by which the injectable drug can be given, such as SC, IM, and/or IV, is printed on the drug label.

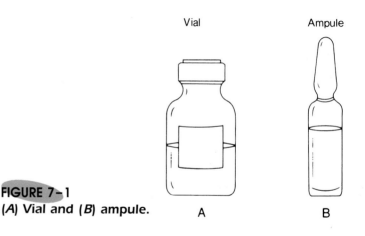

Vial   Ampule

FIGURE 7–1
(A) **Vial and** *(B)* **ampule.**   A   B

Syringes

Types of syringes used for injections include 3-mL and 5-mL calibrated syringes, metal and plastic syringes for prefilled cartridges, tuberculin syringes, and insulin syringes. There are 10-mL, 20-mL, and 50-mL syringes that are used mostly for drug preparations. The syringe is composed of a barrel (outer shell), plunger (inner part), and the tip, where the needle joins the syringe (Fig. 7–2).

PARTS OF A SYRINGE

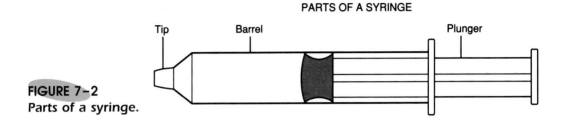

FIGURE 7–2
Parts of a syringe.

Three-Milliliter Syringe

The 3-mL syringe is calibrated in tenths (0.1 mL) and minims (℥). The amount of fluid in the syringe is determined by the rubber end of the plunger that is closest to the tip of the syringe (Fig. 7–3). Remember, milliliter (mL) and cubic centimeter (cc) are used interchangeably.

THREE MILLILITER SYRINGE

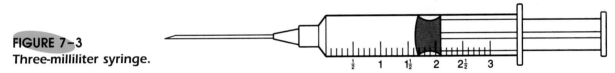

FIGURE 7–3
Three-milliliter syringe.

Five-Milliliter Syringe

The 5-mL syringe is calibrated in 0.2 mL. A 5-mL syringe is usually used when the fluid needed is more than 2½ mL. This syringe is frequently used when reconstituting a dry drug form with sterile water, bacteriostatic water, or saline. Figure 7–4 shows the 5-mL syringe and its markings.

FIVE MILLILITER SYRINGE

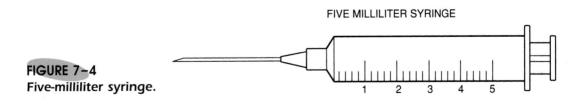

FIGURE 7–4
Five-milliliter syringe.

Tuberculin Syringe

The tuberculin syringe is a 1-mL, slender syringe that is calibrated in tenths (0.1 mL), hundredths (0.01 mL), and minims (Fig. 7–5). This syringe is used when the amount of drug solution to be administered is less than 1 mL and for pediatric and heparin dosages.

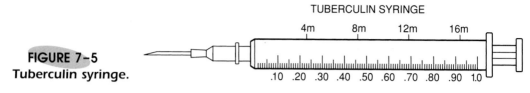

FIGURE 7-5
Tuberculin syringe.

Insulin Syringe

The insulin syringe has a capacity of 1 mL. Insulin is measured in units, and insulin dosage *must NOT* be calculated in milliliters. Insulin syringes are calibrated as 2 units per mark, and 100 units equal 1 mL (Fig. 7–6). *Insulin syringes, NOT tuberculin syringes, must be used for administering insulin.*

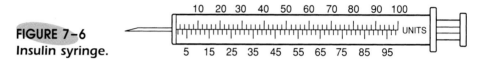

FIGURE 7-6
Insulin syringe.

Prefilled Drug Cartridge and Syringe

Many injectable drugs are packaged in prefilled disposable cartridges. The disposable cartridge is placed into a reusable metal or plastic holder. A prefilled cartridge usually contains 0.1 to 0.2 mL of excess drug solution. Based on the amount of drug to be administered, the excess solution must be expelled prior to administration; check the institution's policy. Figure 7–7 illustrates the Tubex syringe with cartridge. The cartridge can easily be disposed without touching it after use.

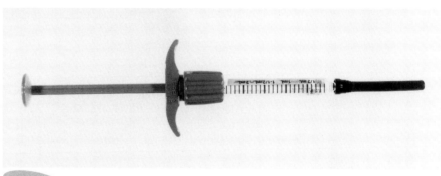

FIGURE 7-7
Tubex syringe with cartridge.
(Courtesy of Wyeth–Ayerst Laboratories, Philadelphia, PA.)

Needles

A needle includes (1) a hub (large metal or plastic part attached to the tip of the syringe), (2) a shaft (thin needle length), and (3) a bevel (end of the needle). Figure 7–8 illustrates the parts of a needle.

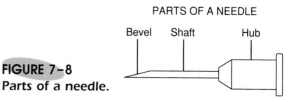

FIGURE 7-8
Parts of a needle.

Needle size is determined by gauge (diameter of the lumen) and by length. The larger the gauge number, the smaller the diameter of the lumen. The smaller the gauge number, the larger the diameter of the lumen. The usual range of needle gauges is from 18 to 26. Needle length varies from ⅜ to 2 inches. Table 7–1 lists the needle sizes and lengths for use in intradermal, subcutaneous, and intramuscular injections.

TABLE 7-1
Needle Size and Length

TYPE OF INJECTION	NEEDLE GAUGE	NEEDLE LENGTHS
Intradermal	25, 26	⅜, ½, ⅝ inches
Subcutaneous	23, 25, 26	⅜, ½, ⅝ inches
Intramuscular	19, 20, 21, 22	1, 1½, 2 inches

When choosing the needle length for an intramuscular injection, the size of the patient and the amount of fatty tissue must be considered. A patient with minimal fatty (subcutaneous) tissue may need a needle length of 1 inch. For an obese patient, the length of the needle for an intramuscular injection may be 1½ to 2 inches.

Insulin syringes and prefilled cartridges have permanently attached needles. With other syringes, needle sizes can be changed. Needle gauge and length are indicated on the syringe package or on the top cover of the syringe. It appears as gauge/length, such as 21g/1½ inch. Figure 7–9 illustrates two combinations of needle gauge and length.

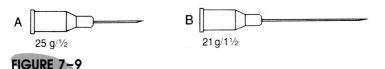

A 25 g/½

B 21 g/1½

FIGURE 7-9
Two combinations of needle gauge and length.

Research has shown that after an injection, medication remains in the hub of the syringe, where the needle joins the syringe. This volume can be as much as 0.2 mL. There is controversy as to whether air should be added to the syringe prior to administration to insure that the total volume is given. The best practice is to follow the institution's policy.

Angles for Injection

For injections, the needle enters the skin at different angles. Intradermal injections are given at a 10- to 15-degree angle, subcutaneous injections at a 45- to 90-degree angle, and intramuscular injections at a 90-degree angle. Figure 7–10 illustrates the angles for intradermal, subcutaneous, and intramuscular injections.

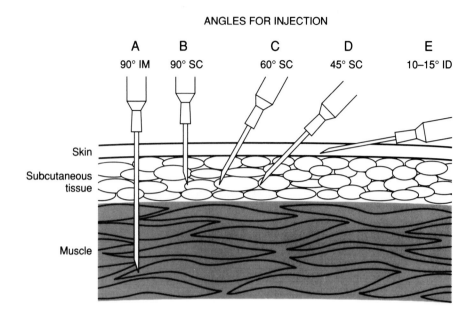

ANGLES FOR INJECTION

Key: A:IM 90°; B, C, D:SC 90°, 60°, 45°;
E:ID (intradermal) 10–15°

FIGURE 7–10
Angles for injection.
(Adapted from Norton, B. A., and Miller, A. M. (1986). *Skills for Professional Nursing Practice.*
Norwalk, CT: Appleton-Century-Crofts. With permission.)

I. Practice Problems: Needles

1. Which would have the larger needle lumen: a 21-gauge needle or a 25-gauge needle? _____

2. Which would have the smaller needle lumen: an 18-gauge needle or a 26-gauge needle? _____

3. Which needle would have a length of 1½ inches: a 20-gauge needle or a 25-gauge needle? _____

4. Which needle would have a length of ⅝ inch: a 21-gauge needle or a 25-gauge needle? _____

5. Which needle would be used for an intramuscular injection: a 21-gauge needle with a 1½-inch length or 25-gauge needle with a ⅝-inch length? _____

INTRADERMAL INJECTIONS

Usually, an intradermal injection is used for skin testing for diagnostic purposes. Primary uses are for tuberculin and allergy testing. The tuberculin syringe (25 g/½ inch) holds 1 mL (16 minims) and is calibrated in 0.1 to 0.01 mL.

The inner aspect of the forearm is often used for diagnostic testing because there is less hair in the area and the test results are easily seen. The upper back can also be used as a testing site. The needle is inserted with the bevel upward at a 10- to 15-degree angle. Do not aspirate. Test results are read 48 to 72 hours after the intradermal injection. A reddened and/or raised area indicates a positive reaction.

SUBCUTANEOUS INJECTIONS

Drugs injected into the subcutaneous (fatty) tissue are absorbed slowly because there are fewer blood vessels in the fatty tissue. The amount of drug solution administered subcutaneously is generally 0.5 to 1 mL at a 45-, 60-, or 90-degree angle. Irritating drug solutions are given intramuscularly because they can cause sloughing of the subcutaneous tissue.

The two types of syringes used for subcutaneous injections are the tuberculin syringe (1 mL), which is calibrated in 0.1 and 0.01 mL, and the 3-mL syringe, which is calibrated in 0.1 mL (Fig. 7–11). The needle gauge commonly used is 25 or 26 gauge, and the length is usually ⅜ to ⅝ inch. Insulin is also administered subcutaneously and is discussed later in this chapter.

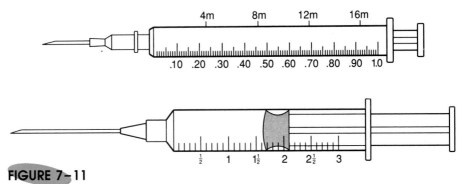

FIGURE 7–11
Syringes used for subcutaneous injections.

Calculation for Subcutaneous Injections

Formulas for solving problems of subcutaneous injections are the basic formula, ratio and proportion, and fractional equation (see Chap. 5). The following problems are examples of injections that can be given subcutaneously.

EXAMPLES

PROBLEM 1: Order: heparin 5000 U, SC.
            Drug available:

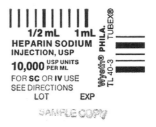

Methods:

Basic formula   Ratio and proportion

$$\frac{D}{H} \times V = \frac{5000}{10,000} \times 1 \text{ or}$$

H	:	V	: :	D	:	X
10,000 U	:	1 mL	: :	5000 U	:	X mL

$$= \frac{5}{10} = 0.5 \text{ mL}$$

$$10,000 \; X = 5000$$

$$X = \frac{5000}{10,000} = \frac{5}{10} =$$
$$0.5 \text{ mL}$$

Answer: Heparin 5000 U = 0.5 mL

PROBLEM 2: Order: morphine 10 mg, SC.
Drug available:

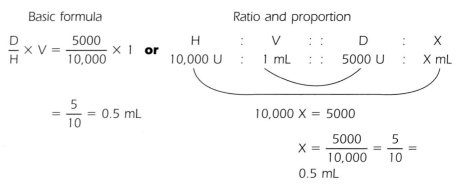

See label with approximate equivalents.

Methods: $\frac{D}{H} \times V = \frac{10}{15} \times 1$ **or**

H	:	V	: :	D	:	X
15 mg	:	1 mL	: :	10 mg	:	X mL

$$= \frac{2}{3} = 0.67 \text{ mL}$$
$$\text{or } 0.7 \text{ mL}$$

$$15 \; X = 10$$

$$X = \frac{\overset{2}{\cancel{10}}}{\underset{3}{\cancel{15}}} = \frac{2}{3} = 0.67 \text{ mL}$$
$$\text{or } 0.7 \text{ mL}$$

Answer: Morphine 10 mg = 0.67 or 0.7 mL (use a tuberculin syringe or a
3-mL syringe).

II. Practice Problems: Subcutaneous injections

Use the formula you chose for calculating oral drug dosages in Chapter 6.

1. Which needle gauge and length should be used for a subcutaneous injection:
a 25 g/⅝ inch or 26 g/⅜ inch? _____

2. Order: heparin 4000 U, SC.
Drug available:

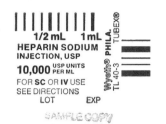

a. How many milliliters of heparin would you give? _____

b. At what angle would you administer the drug? _____

3. Order: heparin 7500 U, SC.
Drug available:

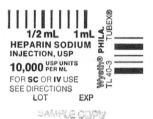

a. How many milliliters of heparin would you give? _____

b. This drug is supplied in a cartridge. What type of syringe should be used? _____

4. Order: atropine SO_4 gr $1/100$, SC.
Drug available:

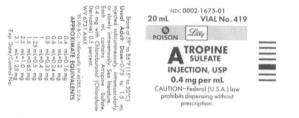

How many milliliters of atropine would you give? _____

5. Order: epinephrine (Adrenalin) 0.35 mg, SC, STAT.
Drug available:

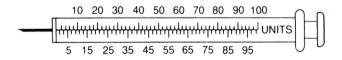

N 0071-3014-09
Adrenalin®
Chloride Solution
(Epinephrine Inhalation
Solution, USP)
10 mg per mL   1:100
For inhalation only
1/4 fl oz (7.5 mL)
Ⓟ **PARKE-DAVIS**

The previous two containers (drug labels) were found in the medicine room. Could either one be used? Explain. _____

INSULIN INJECTIONS

Insulin is prescribed and measured in USP units. Most insulins are manufactured in concentrations of 100 units per mL. Insulin should be administered with an insulin syringe, which is calculated to correspond with the U 100 insulin. Insulin bottles and syringes are color-coded. The U 100 insulin bottle and the U 100 syringe are color-coded orange. Insulin concentrations are also available in U 40 and U 500 but are rarely used. U 40 is being phased out by the U.S. Food and Drug Administration, and U 500 is used mainly in acute situations.

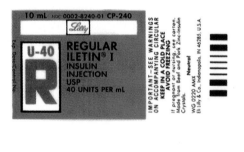

10 mL NDC 0002-8240-01 CP-240
Lilly
U-40
R **REGULAR**
ILETIN® I
INSULIN
INJECTION
USP
40 UNITS PER mL

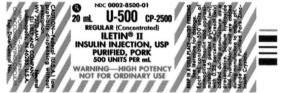

NDC 0002-8500-01
20 mL **U-500** CP-2500
REGULAR (Concentrated)
ILETIN® II
INSULIN INJECTION, USP
PURIFIED, PORK
500 UNITS PER mL
WARNING——HIGH POTENCY
NOT FOR ORDINARY USE

The insulin syringe may be marked on one side in even units (10, 20, 30) and on the other side in odd units (5, 15, 25).

Insulin is easy to prepare and administer as long as the nurse uses the *same insulin concentration with the same calibrated insulin syringe,* e.g., a U 100 insulin bottle and a U 100 insulin syringe. For example, if the prescribed insulin dosage is 30 units, withdraw 30 units from a bottle of U 100 insulin using a U 100-calibrated insulin syringe.

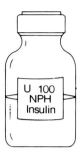

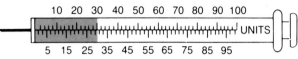

Administering insulin with a tuberculin syringe is *not* suggested and *should be avoided.*

Types of Insulin

Insulin is categorized as fast-acting, intermediate-acting, and long-acting. The following drug labels are arranged according to insulin action.

1. Fast-acting (Humulin R, crystalline (*A*); regular (*B*); and Semilente (*C*))

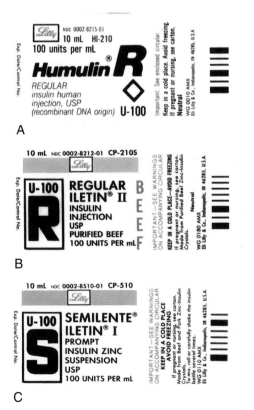

2. Intermediate-acting (Humulin N(*A*), NPH (*B*), and Lente (*C*))

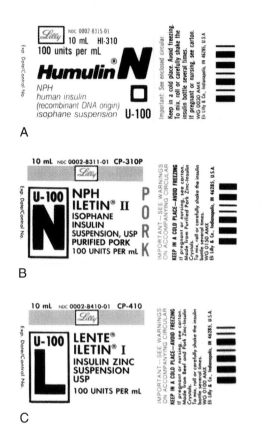

A

B

C

3. Long-acting (PZI (*A*), Ultralente (*B*), and Humulin U (*C*)):

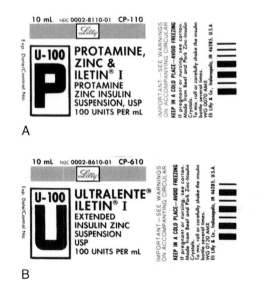

A

B

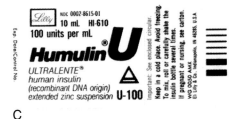

C

Insulins are clear (regular or crystalline insulin) or cloudy (NPH, Lente) because of the substances (protamine and zinc) used to prolong the action of insulin in the body. Only clear (regular) insulin can be given intravenously as well as subcutaneously. Insulin containing protamine and zinc can only be administered subcutaneously.

The sources of insulins are beef, pork, beef–pork, and human (Humulin). Some individuals are allergic to beef insulin, so pork insulin is used because it has biologic properties similar to human insulin.

Insulin is administered subcutaneously at a 45-, 60-, or 90-degree angle into the subcutaneous tissue. The angle for administering insulin depends on the amount of fatty tissue in the patient. For a very thin person, a 45-degree angle is suggested. A 90-degree angle should be used on obese or average-sized persons. When using a 90-degree angle, pinch the skin upward so the insulin is deposited into the fatty tissue.

Mixing Insulins

Regular insulin is frequently mixed with insulins containing protamine, such as NPH, and zinc, such as Lente.

EXAMPLE

Problem and method for mixing insulin.

PROBLEM 1: Order: Regular insulin U-10 and Lente insulin U-40, SC.
Drug available: Regular insulin U-100 and Lente insulin U-100, both in multidose vials. The insulin syringe is marked U-100.

Methods: **1.** Cleanse the rubber tops or diaphragms of insulin bottles.

2. Draw up 40 U of air* and inject into the Lente insulin bottle. Do not allow the needle to come into contact with the Lente insulin solution. Withdraw needle.

3. Draw up 10 U of air and inject into the regular insulin bottle.

4. Withdraw 10 U of regular insulin. Regular insulin is withdrawn before Lente and NPH.

5. Withdraw 40 U of Lente insulin.

---

* You may draw up 50 units of air; inject 40 units into the NPH bottle and 10 units into the regular insulin bottle.

6. Administer the two insulins immediately after mixing. Do not allow the insulin mixture to stand, because unpredicted physical changes might occur. Unpredicted changes are more common with protamine insulins such as NPH and PZI than with Lente insulin.

III. Practice Problems: Insulin

1. Order: NPH insulin 35 U, SC.
Drug available: NPH insulin U 100 and U 100 insulin syringe. Indicate on the insulin syringe the amount of insulin that should be withdrawn.

```
        10  20  30  40  50  60  70  80  90  100
  ╞════╤╤╤╤╤╤╤╤╤╤╤╤╤╤╤╤╤╤╤╤╤╤╤╤╤╤╤╤╤╤╤╤╤╤╤╤╤╤╤╤ UNITS
        5  15  25  35  45  55  65  75  85  95
```

2. Order: Lente insulin 50 U, SC.
Drug available: Lente U 100 and U 100 insulin syringe.
Indicate on the insulin syringe the amount of insulin that should be withdrawn.

```
        10  20  30  40  50  60  70  80  90  100
  ╞════╤╤╤╤╤╤╤╤╤╤╤╤╤╤╤╤╤╤╤╤╤╤╤╤╤╤╤╤╤╤╤╤╤╤╤╤╤╤╤╤ UNITS
        5  15  25  35  45  55  65  75  85  95
```

3. Order: regular insulin U 8 and NPH insulin U 52.
Drug available: regular insulin U 100 and NPH insulin U 100.
The insulin syringe is U 100.
Explain the method for mixing the two insulins.

_____

Mark on the U 100 insulin syringe how much regular insulin should be withdrawn and how much NPH insulin should be withdrawn.

```
        10  20  30  40  50  60  70  80  90  100
  ╞════╤╤╤╤╤╤╤╤╤╤╤╤╤╤╤╤╤╤╤╤╤╤╤╤╤╤╤╤╤╤╤╤╤╤╤╤╤╤╤╤ UNITS
        5  15  25  35  45  55  65  75  85  95
```

4. Order: regular insulin U 15 and Lente insulin U 45.
Drug available: regular insulin U 100 and Lente insulin U 100.
The insulin syringe is U 100.

Explain the method for mixing the two insulins.

_____

Mark on the U 100 insulin syringe how much regular insulin and how much Lente insulin should be withdrawn.

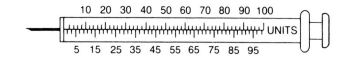

INTRAMUSCULAR INJECTIONS

The IM injection is a common method of administering injectable drugs. The muscle has many blood vessels (more so than fatty tissue), so medications given by intramuscular injections are absorbed more rapidly than those given by SC injections. The volume of solution for an IM injection is 0.5 to 3.0 mL, with the average being 1 to 2 mL. A volume of drug solution greater than 3 mL causes increased muscle tissue displacement and possible tissue damage. Occasionally, 5 mL of certain drugs, such as magnesium sulfate, may be injected in a large muscle, such as the dorsogluteal. Dosages greater than 3 mL are usually divided and given at two different sites.

Needle gauges for IM injections containing thick solutions are 19 and 20, and for thin solutions are 20 to 21. IM injections are administered at a 90-degree angle. The needle length depends on the amount of adipose (fat) and muscle tissues; the average needle length is 1½ inches.

The common sites for IM injections are the deltoid, dorsogluteal, ventrogluteal, and vastus lateralis muscles. Figure 7–12 displays the sites for each muscle used with IM injection. Table 7–2 gives the volume for drug administration, common needle size, client's position, and angle of injection for the four IM injection sites.

TABLE 7–2
Intramuscular Injection Sites in the Adult

	DELTOID	DORSOGLUTEAL	VENTROGLUTEAL	VASTUS LATERALIS
Volume for drug administration	*Usual:* 0.5–1 mL *Maximum:* 2.0 mL	*Usual:* 1.0–3 mL *Maximum:* 3 mL; 5 mL γ-globulin	*Usual:* 1–3 mL *Maximum:* 3–4 mL	*Usual:* 1–3 mL *Maximum:* 3–4 mL
Common needle size	23–25 gauge; ⅝–1½ inches	18–23 gauge; 1¼–3 inches	20–23 gauge; 1¼–2½ inches	20–23 gauge; 1¼–1½ inches
Client's position	Sitting; supine; prone	Prone	Supine; lateral	Sitting (dorsal flex foot); supine
Angle of injection	90° angle, angled slightly toward the acromion	90° angle to flat surface; upper outer quadrant of the buttock *or* outer aspect of line from the posterior iliac crest to the greater trochanter of the femur	80°–90° angle; angle the needle slightly toward the iliac crest	80°–90° angle; thin person: 60°–75° angle

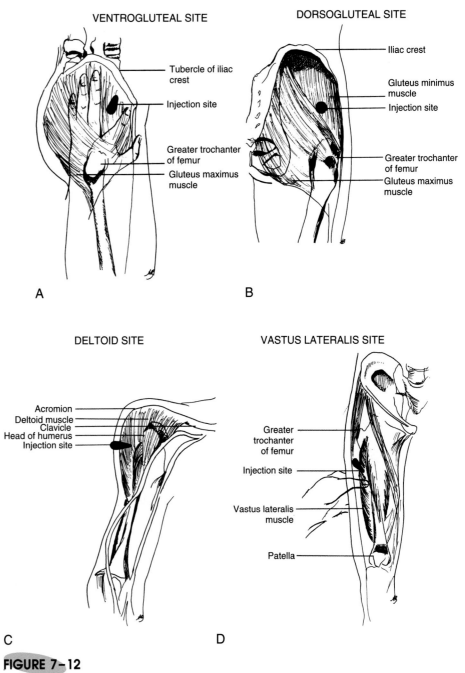

VENTROGLUTEAL SITE

Tubercle of iliac crest

Injection site

Greater trochanter of femur

Gluteus maximus muscle

A

DORSOGLUTEAL SITE

Iliac crest

Gluteus minimus muscle

Injection site

Greater trochanter of femur

Gluteus maximus muscle

B

DELTOID SITE

Acromion
Deltoid muscle
Clavicle
Head of humerus
Injection site

C

VASTUS LATERALIS SITE

Greater trochanter of femur

Injection site

Vastus lateralis muscle

Patella

D

FIGURE 7–12
Intramuscular injection sites.
Source: Kee, J.L., and Hayes, E.R. (1993): *Pharmacology: A Nursing Process Approach,* Philadelphia: W.B. Saunders, pp 34, 35. With permission.

The intramuscular injection section is divided into three subsections: (1) drug solutions for injection, (2) powdered drug reconstitution, and (3) mixing injectable drugs. An example is given for each subsection, and practice problems follow.

Drug Solutions for Injection

Commercially premixed drug solutions are stored in vials and ampules for immediate use. At times, there may be enough drug solution left in a vial for another dose, and the vial may be saved. The balance of a drug solution in an ampule is *always* discarded after the ampule has been opened and used.

EXAMPLES

Two problems are given as examples for calculating IM dosage. Choose one of the four methods for calculating drug dosage.

PROBLEM 1: Order: gentamycin 60 mg, IM.

Drug available: gentamycin 80 mg/2 mL in a vial.

Methods: $\dfrac{D}{H} \times V = \dfrac{60}{80} \times 2$ **or**

$$H \quad : \quad V \quad : : \quad D \quad : \quad X$$
$$80\ mg \quad : \quad 2\ mL \quad : : \quad 60\ mg \quad : \quad X\ mL$$
$$80\ X \quad = \quad 120$$

$$= \dfrac{120}{80} = 1.5\ mL \qquad\qquad X = \dfrac{120}{80} = 1.5\ mL$$

Answer: gentamycin 60 mg = 1.5 mL.

PROBLEM 2: Order: Narcan 0.5 mg, IM, STAT.

Drug available:

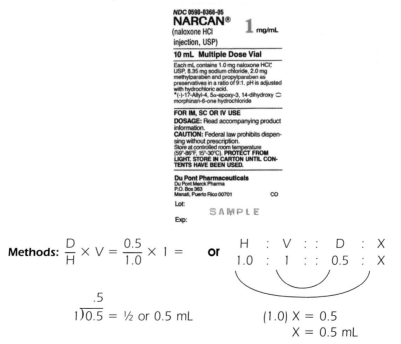

Methods: $\dfrac{D}{H} \times V = \dfrac{0.5}{1.0} \times 1 =$ **or**

$$H \quad : \quad V \quad : : \quad D \quad : \quad X$$
$$1.0 \quad : \quad 1 \quad : : \quad 0.5 \quad : \quad X$$

$$1\overline{)0.5}^{\;.5} = \tfrac{1}{2}\ \text{or}\ 0.5\ mL \qquad\qquad (1.0)\,X = 0.5$$
$$X = 0.5\ mL$$

Answer: Narcan 0.5 mg = 0.5 mL

Powdered Drug Reconstitution

Certain drugs lose their potency in liquid form. Therefore, manufacturers package these drugs in powdered form, and they are reconstituted prior to administration. To reconstitute a drug, look on the drug label or in the instructional insert (circular pamphlet) for the type and amount of diluent to use. Sterile water, bacteriostatic water, and normal saline are the primary diluents. If the type and amount of diluent are not on the drug label or in the instructional insert, call the pharmacy.

The powdered drug occupies space and therefore increases the volume of drug solution. Usually, manufacturers determine the amount of diluent to mix with the drug powder to yield 1 to 2 mL per desired dose. After the powdered drug has been reconstituted, the unused drug solution should be dated, initialed, and refrigerated. Most drugs retain their potency for 48 hours to 1 week when refrigerated. Check the drug circular or drug label for how long the reconstituted drug may be used.

EXAMPLES

PROBLEM 1: Order: oxacillin sodium 500 mg, IM, q6h.
Drug available:

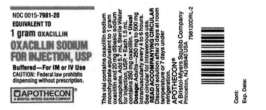

According to the label on the bottle, the amount of powdered drug in the vial is 1 g. The drug label states:
Add 5.7 mL of sterile water (diluent) to the vial. Each 250 mg = 1.5 mL or 1 g = 6 mL.

Methods: Change grams to milligrams or change milligrams to grams (see Table 5–1). 1 gram = 1000 mg *or* 500 mg = 0.500 g (0.5 g). Move the decimal point three spaces to the left.

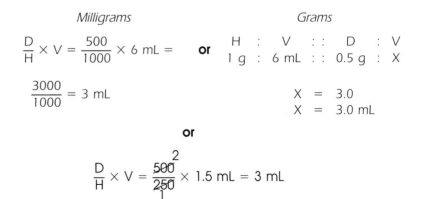

Milligrams	*Grams*

$$\frac{D}{H} \times V = \frac{500}{1000} \times 6\ mL = \quad \textbf{or}$$

$$\frac{3000}{1000} = 3\ mL$$

$$
\begin{array}{ccccccc}
H & : & V & :: & D & : & V \\
1\ g & : & 6\ mL & :: & 0.5\ g & : & X
\end{array}
$$

$$X = 3.0$$
$$X = 3.0\ mL$$

or

$$\frac{D}{H} \times V = \frac{\overset{2}{\cancel{500}}}{\underset{1}{\cancel{250}}} \times 1.5\ mL = 3\ mL$$

Answer: oxacillin sodium 500 mg = 3 mL.

PROBLEM 2: Order: cephapirin (Cefadyl) 250 mg, IM, q6h.

Drug available:

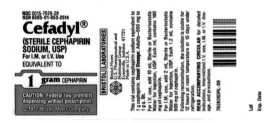

The drug label reads to add 2 mL of sterile or bacterio-static water. Each 1.2 mL contains 500 mg of cephapirin.

Methods: $\dfrac{D}{H} \times V = \dfrac{250}{500} \times 1.2\ \text{mL}$ **or** $\begin{array}{ccccccc} H & : & V & :: & D & : & X \\ 500\ \text{mg} & : & 1.2\ \text{mL} & :: & 250\ \text{mg} & : & X \end{array}$

$$\frac{300}{500} = 500\overline{)300.0}^{\,0.6} \qquad\qquad 500\,X = 300$$

$$X = \frac{300}{500}$$

$$= 0.6\ \text{mL}$$

$$= 0.6\ \text{mL}$$

Answer: cephapirin (Cefadyl) 250 mg = 0.6 mL.

Mixing Injectable Drugs

Drugs mixed together in the same syringe must be compatible to prevent precipitation. To determine drug compatibility, check drug references or check with a pharmacist. When in doubt of compatibility, do *not* mix drugs.

The three methods associated in drug mixing are (1) mixing two drugs in the same syringe from two vials, (2) mixing two drugs in the same syringe from one vial and one ampule, and (3) mixing two drugs in a prefilled cartridge and from a vial.

METHOD 1 Mixing two drugs in the *same syringe* from *two vials*.

1. Draw air into the syringe to equal the amount of solution to be withdrawn from the first vial, and inject the air into the first vial. Do *not* allow the needle to come into contact with the solution. Remove the needle.

2. Draw air into the syringe to equal the amount of solution to be withdrawn from the second vial. Invert second vial and inject the air.

3. Withdraw the desired amount of solution from the second vial.

4. Change the needle unless you will use the entire volume in the first vial.

5. Invert the first vial and withdraw the desired amount of solution.

or

1. Draw air in syringe to equal the amount of solution to be with-drawn and inject the air into the first vial. Withdraw the desired drug dose.

2. Insert a 25-g needle in the rubber-top vial (not in the center) of the second vial. This acts as an air vent. Injecting air into the second vial is *not* necessary.

3. Insert the needle in the center of the rubber-top vial (beside the 25-g needle–air vent), invert the second vial, and withdraw the desired drug dose.

METHOD 2   Mixing two drugs in the same syringe from *one vial and one ampule.*

1. Remove the amount of desired solution from the vial.

2. Aspirate the amount of desired solution from the ampule.

METHOD 3   Mixing two drugs in a *prefilled cartridge from a vial.*

1. Check the drug dose and the amount of solution in the prefilled cartridge. If a smaller dose is needed, expel the excess solution.

2. Draw air into the cartridge to equal the amount of solution to be withdrawn from the vial. Invert the vial and inject the air.

3. Withdraw desired amount of solution from the vial. Make sure the needle remains in the fluid, and do *not* take more solution than needed.

EXAMPLES

Mixing drugs in the same syringe.

PROBLEM 1: Order: meperidine (Demerol) 60 mg and atropine SO$_4$ gr $^1/_{150}$, IM.
The two drugs are compatible.
Drugs available:

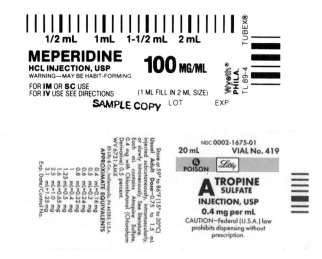

Note: meperidine is in a prefilled Tubex cartridge, and atropine sulfate is in a vial.

How many milliliters of each drug would you give?
Explain how to mix the two drugs.

Methods: Meperidine

$$\frac{D}{H} \times V = \frac{60}{100} \times 1 \quad \textbf{or} \quad \begin{array}{ccccccc} H & : & V & :: & D & : & X \\ 100\ mg & : & 1\ mL & : & 60\ mg & : & X\ mL \end{array}$$

$$= 0.6\ mL \qquad\qquad 100\ X = 60$$
$$X = 0.6\ mL$$

Atropine SO_4

gr $\frac{1}{150}$ = 0.4 mg (see Tables 2–1 and 5–1).

Answer: meperidine (Demerol) 60 mg = 0.6 mL.
atropine gr $\frac{1}{150}$ = 1 mL.

Procedure: Mix two drugs in a cartridge with one drug from a vial.

1. Check drug dose and volume on prefilled cartridge.

2. Expel 0.4 mL and any excess of drug solution from cartridge; 0.6 mL remains in the cartridge.

3. Draw 1 mL of air in the cartridge and inject into the vial.

4. Withdraw 1 mL of atropine from vial into the prefilled cartridge.

PROBLEM 2: Order: meperidine 25 mg, Vistaril 25 mg, and Robinul 0.1 mg, IM. All three drugs are compatible.

Drug available: meperidine (Demerol) is in a 2-mL Tubex cartridge labeled 50 mg/mL. Hydroxyzine (Vistaril) is in a 50 mg/mL ampule. Glycopyrrolate (Robinul) is in a 0.2 mg/mL vial.

How many milliliters of each drug would you give?

_____

Explain how the drugs could be mixed together.

_____

Methods: a. meperidine 25 mg. Label: 50 mg/mL.

$$\frac{D}{H} \times V = \frac{25}{50} \times 1 \quad \textbf{or} \quad \begin{array}{ccccccc} H & : & V & :: & D & : & X \\ 50\ mg & : & 1\ mL & : & 25\ mg & : & X\ mL \end{array}$$

$$= 0.5\ mL \qquad\qquad 50\ X = 25$$
$$X = \text{½ mL or 0.5 mL}$$

b. Vistaril 25 mg. Label: 50 mg/mL ampule.

$$\frac{D}{H} \times V = \frac{25}{50} \times 1 \quad \textbf{or} \quad \begin{array}{ccccccc} H & : & V & :: & D & : & X \\ 50\ mg & : & 1\ mL & : & 25\ mg & : & X\ mL \end{array}$$

$$= 0.5\ mL \qquad\qquad 50\ X = 25$$
$$X = \text{½ mL or 0.5 mL}$$

c. Robinul 0.1 mg. Label: 0.2 mg/mL.

$$\frac{D}{H} \times V = \frac{0.1}{0.2} \times 1 \quad \textbf{or}$$

$$= 0.5 \text{ mL}$$

H : V : : D : X
0.2 mg : 1 mL : : 0.1 mg : X mL

0.2 X = 0.1
X = 0.5 mL

Answer: meperidine (Demerol) 25 mg = 0.5 mL; Vistaril 25 mg = 0.5 mL; Robinul 0.1 mg = 0.5 mL.

Procedure: Mix three drugs in the cartridge.

1. Check drug dose and volume on prefilled cartridge. Expel 0.5 mL of meperidine and any excess of drug solution from cartridge.

2. Draw 0.5 mL of air into the cartridge and inject into the vial containing the Robinul.

3. Withdraw 0.5 mL of Robinul from the vial into the prefilled cartridge containing meperidine.

4. Withdraw 0.5 mL of Vistaril from the ampule into the cartridge.

IV. Practice Problems: Intramuscular Injections

1. Order: tobramycin (Nebcin) 50 mg, IM, q8h.
Drug available:

NDC 0002-1499-01
2 mL VIAL No. 781
Ⓡ *Lilly*
NEBCIN®
TOBRAMYCIN
SULFATE
INJECTION
USP
Equiv. to Tobramycin
80 mg per 2 mL
Multiple Dose
For I.M. or I.V. Use
Must dilute for I.V. use.
ELI LILLY AND COMPANY
Indianapolis, IN 46285, U.S.A.
WW 1440 AMX
Exp. Date/Control No.

How many mL of tobramycin would you give? _____

2. Order: methylprednisolone (Solu-Medrol) 75 mg, IM, qd.
Drug available: 125 mg/2 mL in vial.
How many mL would you give? _____

3. Order: vitamin B$_{12}$ (cyanocobalamin) 30 mcg (μg), IM, qd.
Drug available:

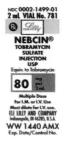

TUBEX® TL 37-3
1/2 mL   1 mL
CYANOCOBALAMIN
INJECTION, USP
VITAMIN B12
100 MCG PER ML
FOR **SC, IM** OR **IV** USE
LOT   EXP
SAMPLE COPY
Wyeth® PHILA.

How many mL of cyanocobalamin would you give? _____

4. Order: Narcan 0.2 mg, IM, STAT.
Drug available:

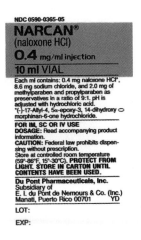

How many mL would you give? _____

5. Order: droperidol 5 mg, IM, 1 hour prior to surgery.
Drug available:

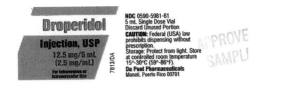

How many mL should be given 1 hour prior to surgery? _____

6. Order: haloperidol (Haldol) 4 mg, IM, q8h.
Drug available:

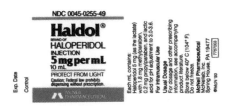

How many mL should the patient receive? _____

7. Order: secobarbital (Seconal) 125 mg, IM, 1 hour prior to surgery.
Drug available: Seconal 50 mg/mL.
How many mL would you give? _____

8. Order: Thiamine HCl 75 mg, IM, qd.
Drug available: 100 and 200 mg/mL vials.
  a. Which vial would you use? _____
  b. How many mL would you give? _____

9. Order: hydroxyzine (Vistaril) 25 mg, deep IM, STAT.
Drug available: Vistaril 100 mg/2 mL in a vial.
How many mL would you give? _____

10. Order: clindamycin 0.3 g, IM, q6h.
Drug available:

> STERILE   NDC 0205-2801-26   Control   Exp.
> **Clindamycin Phosphate Injection, USP**
> **300 mg** Equivalent to
> 300 mg clindamycin.   22438 D51
> WARNING: If given intravenously, LEDERLE
> must be diluted before use.   PARENTERALS, INC.
>   Carolina,
> **2 mL Single Dose Vial**   Puerto Rico 00630

Change gram to milligrams (3 spaces to the right) or milligrams to
gram (3 spaces to the left).
0.300 g = 300 mg (the label is in milligrams)

How many mL should be given? _____

11. Order: meperidine (Demerol) 35 mg and promethazine (Phenergan) 10 mg, IM.
Drugs available: meperidine 50 mg/mL in a prefilled cartridge
that holds 2 mL of solution (2-mL cartridge); promethazine 25 mg/
mL in an ampule.

> | 1/2 mL   1 mL   1-1/2 mL   2 mL | TUBEX®
> **MEPERIDINE**
> HCL INJECTION, USP   **50 MG/ML**
> WARNING—MAY BE HABIT-FORMING
> FOR **IM** OR **SC** USE   Wyeth®
> FOR **IV** USE SEE DIRECTIONS   (1 ML FILL IN 2 ML SIZE)   PHILA.
>   LOT   EXP   TL 87-4
>   **SAMPLE COPY**

a. How many mL of meperidine would you give? _____
b. How many mL of promethazine would you give? _____
c. Explain how the two drugs would be mixed in the cartridge.

_____

12. Order: meperidine (Demerol) 50 mg and atropine SO$_4$ 0.3 mg, IM.
Drugs available:

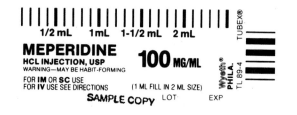

> | 1/2 mL   1 mL   1-1/2 mL   2 mL | TUBEX®
> **MEPERIDINE**
> HCL INJECTION, USP   **100 MG/ML**
> WARNING—MAY BE HABIT-FORMING
> FOR **IM** OR **SC** USE   Wyeth®
> FOR **IV** USE SEE DIRECTIONS   (1 ML FILL IN 2 ML SIZE)   PHILA.
>   **SAMPLE COPY** LOT   EXP   TL 89-4

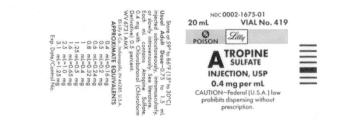

a. How many mL of meperidine would you give? _____

b. How many mL of atropine would you give? _____

c. Explain how the two drugs are mixed in the cartridge.

_____

13. Order: procaine penicillin G (Wycillin) 400,000 U, IM, q12h.
Drug available:

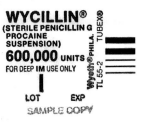

600,000 U = 1 mL.
How many mL of procaine penicillin would you withdraw? _____

14. Order: heparin 2500 U, SC, q6h.
Drug available:

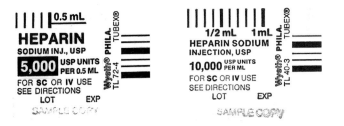

a. Which drug cartridge would you use? _____

b. How many mL of heparin would you give? _____

15. Order: chlordiazepoxide HCl (Librium) 50 mg, IM, STAT.
Drug available: 5 mL of dry Librium (100 mg) powder in ampule.
Add 2 mL of special intramuscular diluent to the ampule. When
diluted, the powder content may increase the volume.

How many mL would be equivalent to 50 mg? _____
Explain. _____

16. Order: cefamandole (Mandol) 500 mg, IM, q6h.
Drug available:

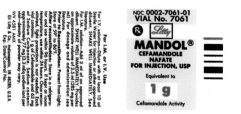

a. Change milligrams to grams (see Chap. 1).

_____

b. How many mL of diluent would you add (see drug label)?

_____

c. What size syringe would you use? _____

d. How many mL = 1 g; how many mL = 500 mg? _____

17. Order: ampicillin (Polycillin-N) 400 mg, IM, q6h.
Drug available:

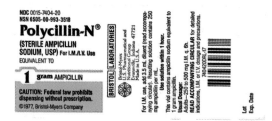

Drug label reads to add 3.5 mL of diluent. Total volume of solution would = 4.0 mL (1 g = 4 mL).

How many mL of ampicillin should be withdrawn? _____

18. Order: morphine gr ⅙, IM, STAT.
Drug available:

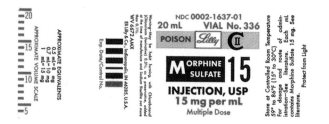

Change grains to milligrams (see Chap. 1 or Tables 2–1 and 5–1).
How many mL of morphine would you give? _____

19. Order: cephradine (Velosef) 250 mg, IM, q6h.
(give 250 mg = 2 mL)
Drug available:

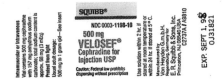

How much diluent would you add to the vial for 2 mL of Velosef 250 mg? _____

20. Order: ampicillin 0.25 g, IM, q6h.
Drug available:

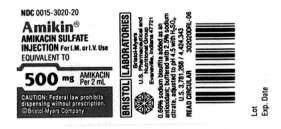

a. To change grams to milligrams, move the decimal point 3 spaces to the _____
b. How many mL of diluent would you add to the vial? _____
c. How many mL should the patient receive? _____

Questions 21 through 23 relate to drug dosage per body weight.

21. Order: amikacin (Amikin) 15 mg/kg/day, q8h, IM.
Drug available:

Patient weighs 140 pounds.

a. How many kilograms does the patient weigh? _____
b. How many milligrams should the patient receive daily? _____
c. How many milligrams should the patient receive q8h (three divided doses)? _____
d. How many mL should the patient receive q8h? _____

22. Order: netilmicin SO_4 (Netromycin) 2.0 mg/kg, q8h, IM.
The patient weighs 174 pounds.
Drug available: netilmicin 100 mg/mL.

    a. How many kilograms does the patient weigh? _____

    b. How many milligrams should the patient receive daily? _____

    c. How many milligrams should the patient receive q8h? _____

    d. How many mL should the patient receive q8h? _____

23. Order: kanamycin (Kantrex) 15 mg/kg/day, q12h.
Drug available: (drug is also available in 1 g = 3 mL vial).

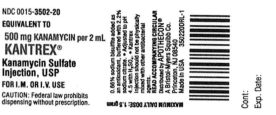

Patient weighs 67 kg.

    a. How many milligrams should the patient receive per day? _____

    b. How many milligrams should the patient receive every 12 hours? _____

    c. How many mL should the patient receive per dose? _____

    d. How many mL from the 1 g = 3 mL vial should the patient receive per dose? _____

Questions 24 through 28 relate to dimensional analysis. Refer to Chapter 5.

24. Order: droperidol 2 mg, IM, STAT.

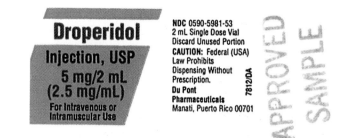

Factors: 5 mg/2 mL; 2 mg/1
Conversion factor: *none*; order and drug available are both in milligrams.
How many mL of droperidol should be given? _____

25. Order: codeine gr ½, IM, PRN.
Drug available:

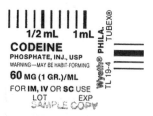

Factors: 60 mg = 1 mL
gr ½/1
Conversion factor: 1 gr = 60 mg
How many milliliters of codeine would you give? _____

26. Order: cephapirin (Cefadyl) 500 mg, IM, q6h.
Drug available:

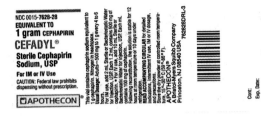

How many mL of diluent would you add? _____
Cefadyl 1 g = _____ mL; 500 mg = _____ mL
Factors: 1 g/_____ mL; 500 mg/1
Conversion factor: 1 g = 1000 mg
How many milliliters of Cefadyl would you give? _____

27. Order: methicillin (Staphcillin) 500 mg, IM, q8h.
Drug available:

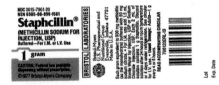

a. Factors (drug label and drug order): _____
b. Conversion factor: _____
c. How many mL of Staphcillin would you give? _____

28. Order: cefazolin (Ancef) 0.25 g, IM, q 12h.
Drug available:

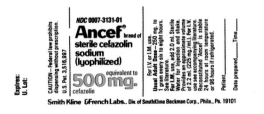

Note: Change grams to milligrams; drug label is in milligrams.

a. Label states to add _____ mL or _____ diluent.
b. How many mL of Ancef would you give? _____

DIRECT INTRAVENOUS INJECTIONS

Medications that are given by the IV injection route are calculated in the same manner as medications for IM injection. This route often is referred to as IV push. Clinically, it is the preferred route for patients with poor muscle mass, decreased circulation, or when the drug is poorly absorbed from the tissues. Medications administered by this route have a rapid onset of action, and calculation errors can have serious, even fatal consequences. Drug literature must be read carefully and attention paid to the amount of drug that can be given per minute. If the drug is pushed into the bloodstream at a faster rate than specified in the drug literature, adverse reactions to the medication are likely to occur.

Calculating the amount of time needed to infuse a drug given by direct IV infusion can be determined by using ratio and proportion.

EXAMPLES

Set up a ratio and proportion using the recommended amount of drug per minute on one side of the equation; these are the known variables. On the other side of the equation are the desired amount of drug and unknown desired minutes.

PROBLEM 1: Order: Dilantin 200 mg, IV, STAT.
Drug available: Dilantin 250 mg/5 mL. IV infusion not to exceed 50 mg/minute.

known drug : known minutes : : desired drug : desired minutes
$$50 \text{ mg} : 1 \text{ min} : : 200 \text{ mg} : X$$
$$50 X = 200$$
$$X = 4 \text{ minutes}$$

PROBLEM 2: Order: Lasix 120 mg, IV, STAT.
Drug available: Lasix 10 mg/mL. IV infusion not to exceed 40 mg/minute.

known drug : known minutes : : desired drug : desired minutes
$$40 \text{ mg} : 1 \text{ min} : : 120 \text{ mg} : X$$
$$40 X = 120$$
$$X = 3 \text{ minutes}$$

V. Practice Problems: Direct IV Injection

1. Order: protamine sulfate 50 mg, IV, STAT.
Drug available: protamine sulfate 50 mg/10 mL. IV infusion not to exceed 5 mg/minute.

2. Order: dextrose 50% in 50 mL, IV, STAT.
Drug available: dextrose 50% in 50 mL. IV infusion not to exceed 10 mL/minute.

3. Order: calcium gluconate 4.5 mEq, IV, STAT. IV infusion not to exceed 1.5 mL/minute. Note: 4.65 mEq/10 mL.

Drug available:

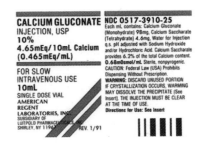

4. Order: prednisolone 50 mg, IV, q12h.
Drug available: prednisolone 50 mg in 5 mL. IV infusion not to exceed 10 mg/minute.

5. Order: morphine sulfate 6 mg, IV, q3h, PRN.
Drug available: morphine sulfate 10 mg/mL. Infusion not to exceed 10 mg/4 minutes.

6. Order: digoxin 0.25 mg, IV, qd. Infuse slowly over 5 minutes.
How many mL/min should be infused?
Drug available:

DIGOXIN **0.5** MG
INJECTION, USP PER TUBEX
(0.25 MG PER ML)

1/2 mL   1mL   1-1/2 mL   2 mL

Wyeth®
PHILA.
FOR IM
OR IV USE

TUBEX®

TL 112-4

SAMPLE COPY   LOT   EXP

7. Order: Haldol 2 mg, IV, q4h, PRN. IV infusion not to exceed 1 mg/minute.
Drug available:

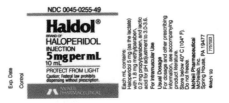

8. Order: Ativan 6 mg, IV, q6h, PRN.
Drug available: Ativan 4 mg/mL. IV infusion not to exceed 2 mg/minute.

NOTE

When a drug is being pushed through IV tubing, the type of fluid used for infusion must be compatible with the drug or precipitation can result. Incompatibilities can be avoided if IV tubing is flushed with a drug-compatible solution, either sterile normal saline or sterile water, prior to and after administration.

ANSWERS

I. Needles

1. The 21-gauge needle, because it is the smaller gauge number.
2. The 26-gauge needle, because it is the larger gauge number.
3. The 20-gauge needle, because it has the larger lumen (small gauge). A needle with a 20 gauge and 1½-inch length is used for IM injection.
4. The 25-gauge needle, because it has the smaller lumen (larger gauge). It is used for SC injections. The length of the needle is not long enough for an IM injection.
5. The 21-gauge needle with 1½-inch length (21 g/1½ inch). Muscle is under subcutaneous or fatty tissue, so a longer needle size is needed.

II. Subcutaneous Injections

1. *Both* needle gauge and length combinations could be used.
2. a. 0.4 mL   **b.** 45- to 60-degree angle. The angle depends on the amount of fatty tissue in the patient.
3. a. ¾ mL or 0.75 mL   **b.** Tubex syringe, a reusable plastic or metal syringe.
4. Change grains (apothecary system) to milligrams (metric system). See Table 2–1. gr $\frac{1}{100}$ = 0.6 mg.

$$\frac{D}{H} \times V = \frac{0.6}{0.4} \times 1 \quad \textbf{or} \qquad
\begin{array}{ccccccc}
H & : & V & : : & D & : & X \\
0.4 \text{ mg} & : & 1 \text{ mL} & : : & 0.6 \text{ mg} & : & X \text{ mL}
\end{array}$$

$$\qquad\qquad\qquad\qquad\qquad 0.4 = 0.6$$

$$= \frac{0.6}{0.4} = 1.5 \text{ mL} \qquad\qquad X = \frac{0.6}{0.4} = 1.5 \text{ mL}$$

5. *No.* One drug is for topical use, and the other drug, with decreased strength (1 : 100), is for inhalation only.

III. Insulin

1. Withdraw 35 U of NPH insulin to the 35 mark on the insulin syringe. Both the insulin and the syringe have the same concentration: U 100.

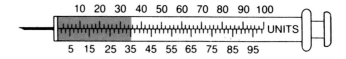

2. Withdraw 50 U of Lente insulin to the 50 mark on the insulin syringe. Both the insulin and the syringe have the same concentration: U 100.

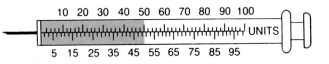

3. Inject 52 U of air into the NPH insulin bottle. Do not allow the needle to touch the insulin solution. Inject 8 U of air into the regular insulin bottle, and withdraw 8 U of regular insulin. Withdraw 52 U of NPH insulin. Total amount of insulin should be 60 U. Do *not* allow the insulin mixture to stand. Administer immediately, because NPH contains protamine, and unpredicted physical changes could result.

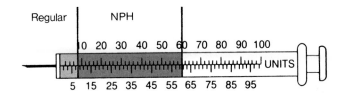

4. Inject 45 U of air into the Lente insulin bottle. Inject 15 U of air into the regular insulin bottle, and withdraw 15 U of regular insulin. Withdraw 45 U of Lente insulin. Total amount of insulin should be 60 U. Insulin mixture can stand for a short period of time because it is Lente insulin.

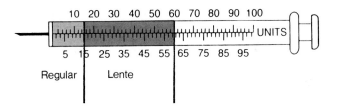

IV. Intramuscular Injections

1. $\dfrac{D}{H} \times V = \dfrac{50}{80} \times 2 \text{ mL}$ **or**

$$\begin{array}{ccccccc} H & : & V & : : & D & : & X \\ 80 \text{ mg} & : & 2 \text{ mL} & : : & 50 \text{ mg} & : & X \text{ mL} \end{array}$$

$$= \dfrac{100}{80} = 1.25 \text{ mL}$$

$$80 X = 100$$
$$X = \dfrac{100}{80} = 1.25 \text{ mL}$$

Answer: tobramycin 50 mg = 1.25 mL

2. $\dfrac{D}{H} \times V = \dfrac{\overset{3}{\cancel{75}}}{\underset{5}{\cancel{125}}} \times 2 \text{ mL}$ **or**

$$\begin{array}{ccccccc} H & : & V & : : & D & : & X \\ 125 \text{ mg} & : & 2 \text{ mL} & : : & 75 \text{ mg} & : & X \text{ mL} \end{array}$$

$$= \dfrac{6}{5} = 1.2 \text{ mL}$$

$$125 X = 150$$
$$X = 1.2 \text{ mL}$$

Answer: methylprednisolone 75 mg = 1.2 mL

3. 0.3 mL of vitamin B_{12} (cyanocobalamin)

4. 0.5 mL of Narcan

5. $\dfrac{D}{H} \times V = \dfrac{5}{12.5} \times 5 =$ **or**

$$\dfrac{25}{12.5} = 2 \text{ mL of droperidol}$$

H	:	V	: :	D	:	X
12.5 mg	:	5 mL	: :	5 mg	:	X

$$12.5\,X = 25$$
$$X = 2 \text{ mL}$$

6. $\dfrac{D}{H} \times V = \dfrac{4}{5} \times 1 = \dfrac{4}{5}$ **or**

H	:	V	: :	D	:	X
5 mg	:	1 mL	: :	4 mg	:	X

0.8 mL of Haldol

$$5\,X = 4 = 0.8 \text{ mL}$$
$$X = 0.8 \text{ mL}$$

7. 2.5 mL of secobarbital

8. a. 100 mg vial
   b. 0.75 mL of thiamine

9. ½ or 0.5 mL of hydroxyzine

10. 0.300 g = 300 mg

$$\dfrac{D}{H} \times V = \dfrac{\cancel{300}^{1}}{\cancel{300}_{1}} \times 2 \text{ mL} = 2 \text{ mL of clindamycin}$$

11. a. meperidine 35 mg = 0.7 mL
   b. promethazine 10 mg = 0.4 mL
   c. Procedure: **1.** Check meperidine dose and volume in prefilled cartridge.
          2. Expel 0.3 mL and any excess in prefilled cartridge; 0.7 mL of solution should remain.
          3. Withdraw 0.4 mL of promethazine from ampule into cartridge.

12. a. meperidine 50 mg = ½ or 0.5 mL
   b. atropine 0.3 mg = 0.75 or 0.8 mL
   Atropine:

$$\dfrac{D}{H} \times V = \dfrac{0.3}{0.4} \times 1 \text{ mL} \quad \textbf{or}$$

H	:	V	: :	D	:	X
0.4 mg	:	1 mL	: :	0.3 mg	:	X mL

$$\begin{array}{r} 0.75 \\ 0.4\overline{)0.3\,00} \end{array} = 0.75 \text{ or } 0.8 \text{ mL}$$

$$0.4\,X = 0.3$$
$$X = \dfrac{0.3}{0.4} = 0.75 \text{ or } 0.8 \text{ mL}$$

   c. 1. Both drugs are compatible.
       2. Prefilled cartridge contains 100 mg = 1 mL. Expel 0.5 mL and any excess in the prefilled cartridge; 0.5 mL drug remains.
       3. Inject 0.75 (0.8) mL of air into the vial, and withdraw the same amount of atropine into the cartridge.

13. $\dfrac{D}{H} \times V = \dfrac{400,000}{600,000} \times 1 \text{ mL}$ **or**

H	:	V	: :	D	:	X
600,000 U	:	1 mL	: :	400,000 U	:	X mL

$$= \dfrac{4}{6} = 0.66 \text{ or } 0.7 \text{ mL}$$

$$600,000\,X = 400,000$$
$$X = 0.66 \text{ or } 0.7 \text{ mL}$$

Answer: procaine penicillin U 400,000 = 0.7 mL

14. a. Use either heparin cartridge: 5000 U/0.5 mL or 10,000 U/1 mL.
   b. 0.25 mL of heparin

15. Librium 50 mg = 1 mL (100 mg = 2 mL)
After adding 2 mL of diluent, withdraw the entire drug solution to determine the total volume of drug solution. Expel half of the solution; the remaining drug solution is equivalent to chlordiazepoxide (Librium) 50 mg.

16. a. Change milligrams to grams (smaller to larger number) by moving the decimal point three spaces to the *left*. 500. mg = 0.5 g. Because the drug weight on the label is in grams, the conversion is to grams. However, the drug can be converted to milligrams by changing grams to milligrams (moving the decimal point three spaces to the *right*): 1 g = 1.000 mg = 1000 mg.

  b. Drug label states to add 3 mL of diluent and, after reconstituted, the drug solution will be 3.5 mL. Mandol 1 g = 3.5 mL.

  c. A 5-mL syringe is preferred: however, a 3-mL syringe can be used because less than 3 mL of the drug solution is needed.

  d. $\dfrac{D}{H} \times V = \dfrac{0.5}{1} \times 3.5$ mL   **or**

$$H \quad : \quad V \quad :: \quad D \quad : \quad X$$
$$1000 \text{ mg} : 3.5 \text{ mL} :: 500 \text{ mg} : X \text{ mL}$$

$= 1.75$ or 1.8 mL

$$1000\ X = 1750$$
$$X = 1.75 \text{ or } 1.8 \text{ mL}$$

Answer: cefamandole (Mandol) 500 mg = 1.8 mL

17. Change 400 milligrams to grams.

$$400 \text{ mg} = .400 \text{ g or } 0.4 \text{ g}$$

$\dfrac{D}{H} \times V = \dfrac{0.4}{1} \times 4$ **or**

$$H \quad : \quad V \quad :: \quad D \quad : \quad X$$
$$1 \text{ g} \quad : \quad 4 \text{ mL} \quad :: \quad 0.4 \text{ g} \quad : \quad X \text{ mL}$$

$= 1.6$ mL

$$X = 4 \times 0.4$$
$$X = 1.6 \text{ mL}$$

Ampicillin 400 mg or 0.4 g = 1.6 mL

18. 1 gr = 60 mg; gr ⅙ = 10 mg

$\dfrac{D}{H} \times V = \dfrac{\overset{2}{\cancel{10}}}{\underset{3}{\cancel{15}}} \times 1$ mL   **or**

$$H \quad : \quad V \quad :: \quad D \quad : \quad X$$
$$15 \text{ mg} : 1 \text{ mL} :: 10 \text{ mg} : X \text{ mL}$$

$= \dfrac{2}{3} = 0.66$ or 0.7 mL

$$15\ X = 10$$
$$X = 0.66 \text{ or } 0.7 \text{ mL}$$

19. 4 mL of diluent

20. a. right, 0.25 g = 250 mg
  b. 1.8 mL (after dilution, 2 mL)
  c. 1 mL = 250 mg of ampicillin

21. a. 140 ÷ 2.2 = 63.6 kg
  b. 15 mg × 63.6 × 1 = 954 mg daily
  c. 954 ÷ 3 = 318 mg of amikacin q8h

  d. $\dfrac{D}{H} \times V = \dfrac{318}{500} \times 2$ **or**

$$H \quad : \quad V \quad :: \quad D \quad : \quad X$$
$$500 \text{ mg} : 2 \text{ mL} :: 318 \text{ mg} : X \text{ mL}$$

$= \dfrac{636}{500} = 1.27$ or 1.3 mL

$$500\ X = 636$$
$$X = 1.27 \text{ or } 1.3 \text{ mL}$$

Answer: give 1.27 or 1.3 mL of amikacin q8h (three times a day).

22. a. $174 \div 2.2 = 79.1$ kg
    b. 2 mg $\times$ 79.1 = 158 mg daily
    c. $158 \div 3 = 52$ mg or 50 mg q8h

    d. $\dfrac{D}{H} \times V = \dfrac{\overset{5}{\cancel{50}}}{\underset{10}{\cancel{100}}} \times 1$ mL   **or**   H : V :: D : X
                                       100 mg : 1 mL :: 50 mg : X mL

                  $= \dfrac{5}{10} = 0.5$ mL   100 X = 50
                                              X = 0.5 mL

                          Answer: netilmicin 50 mg = 0.5 mL

23. a. 15 mg/67 kg/day = 15 $\times$ 67 = 1005 mg/day.
    b. 500 mg (1005 mg $\div$ 2 = 500 mg)

    c. $\dfrac{\overset{1}{\cancel{500}}}{\underset{1}{\cancel{500}}} \times 2 = 2$ mL per dose of Kantrex

    d. 1 g = 1000 mg $\dfrac{D}{H} \times V = \dfrac{\overset{1}{\cancel{500}}}{\underset{2}{\cancel{1000}}} \times 3 = \dfrac{3}{2} = 1.5$ mL

24. milliliters $= \dfrac{2 \text{ mL} \times 2 \cancel{mg}}{5 \cancel{mg} \times 1} = \dfrac{4}{5} = 0.8$ mL

    0.8 mL of droperidol

25. milliliters $= \dfrac{1 \text{ mL} \times \cancel{60} \cancel{mg} \times 0.5 \cancel{gr}}{\cancel{60} \cancel{mg} \times 1 \cancel{gr} \times 1} = 0.5$ mL

26. a. 2 mL of diluent (sterile or bacteriostatic water)
    b. 1 g = 2.4; 500 mg = 1.2 mL (as stated on the label)
    c. Factors: 1 g/2.4 mL; 500 mg/1

    d. milliliters $= \dfrac{2.4 \times 1 \cancel{g} \times \overset{1}{\cancel{500}} \cancel{mg}}{1 \cancel{g} \times \underset{2}{\cancel{1000}} \cancel{mg} \times 1} = \dfrac{2.4}{2} = 1.2$ mL

    Give 1.2 mL of Cefadyl.

27. a. Factors: drug label: 1 g/2 mL
                    drug order: 500 mg/1
    b. Conversion factor: 1 g = 1000 mg

    c. milliliters $= \dfrac{2 \text{ mL} \times 1 \cancel{g} \times \overset{1}{\cancel{500}} \cancel{mg}}{1 \cancel{g} \times \underset{2}{\cancel{1000}} \cancel{mg} \times 1} = \dfrac{2}{2} = 1$ mL

28. 0.25 g = 0.025 mg (250 mg)

    a. Drug label: add 2 mL diluent = 2.2 mL of drug solution.
    b. Give 1.1 mL of Ancef.

V. Direct IV Injection

1. known drug : known minutes : : desired drug : desired minutes
                5 mg : 1 min : : 50 mg : X
                      5 X = 50
                        X = 10 minutes

2. known drug : known minutes : : desired drug : desired minutes
                10 mL : 1 min : : 50 mL : X
                     10 X = 50
                      X = 5 minutes

3. known drug : known minutes : : desired drug : desired minutes
1.5 mL : 1 min : : 10 mL : X
1.5 X = 10
X = 6.6 minutes or 7 minutes

4. known drug : known minutes : : desired drug : desired minutes
10 mg : 1 min : : 50 mg : X
10 X = 50
X = 5 minutes

5. known drug : known minutes : : desired drug : desired minutes
10 mg : 4 min : : 6 mg : X
10 X = 24
X = 2.4 minutes

6. known drug : known minutes : : desired drug : desired minutes
1 mL : 5 min : : X mL : 1 min
5 X = 1
X = 0.2 mL/minute

7. known drug : known minutes : : desired drug : desired minutes
1 mg : 1 min : : 2 mg : X
X = 2 minutes

8. known drug : known minutes : : desired drug : desired minutes
2 mg : 1 min : : 6 mg : X
2X = 6
X = 3 minutes

Intravenous Preparations with Clinical Applications

OBJECTIVES

- Name catheter sites for intravenous access.
- Examine the three methods for calculating intravenous (IV) flow rate and select one of the methods for IV calculation.
- Calculate drops per minute of prescribed IV solutions for IV therapy.
- Determine the drop factor according to the manufacturer's product specification.
- Calculate the drug dosage for IV medications.
- Calculate the flow rate for IV drugs being administered in a prescribed amount of solution.
- Explain the types and uses of electronic IV delivery devices.

Intravenous (IV) therapy is used for administering fluids containing water, dextrose, vitamins, electrolytes, and drugs. Approximately 90% of all hospitalized patients, some outpatients, and some home-care patients receive IV therapy. Drugs are administered intravenously for direct absorption and fast action. There are many drugs that cannot be absorbed through the gastrointestinal tract, and the IV route provides bioavailability. Many drugs administered IV are irritating to the veins because of the drug's pH or osmolality and must be diluted and administered slowly.

Advantages of IV drug therapy are (1) rapid drug distribution into the bloodstream, (2) rapid onset of action, and (3) no drug loss to tissues. There are many disadvantages of IV therapy, some of which are sepsis, thrombosis, phlebitis, air emboli, infiltration, and extravasation. The nurse must monitor for signs of these complications during the course of IV therapy.

Two methods are used to administer IV fluid and drugs: (1) continuous IV infusion and (2) intermittent IV fusion. Continuous IV administration replaces fluid loss, maintains fluid balance, and is a vehicle for drug administration. Intermittent IV administration is primarily used for giving IV drugs.

Nurses play an important role in preparing and administering IV solutions and drugs. Nursing functions and responsibilities include (1) knowledge of intravenous sets and their drop factors, (2) calculating IV flow rates, (3) mixing drugs and diluting in IV solution, (4) regulating IV infusion devices, and (5) maintaining patency of IV accesses.

INTRAVENOUS ACCESS SITES

The successful administration of IV drugs and fluids is dependent on a patent IV access. The most common site is the peripheral site, where a short catheter or needle is inserted in a vein in the hand or arm. Feet and legs can be used, but the risk of a deep vein thrombus is always present. For individuals without adequate peripheral sites or those requiring long term IV therapy, a central venous site is chosen. Central venous sites are the superior vena cava and the inferior vena cava. The superior vena cava is accessed from the internal jugular vein and the right or left subclavian vein, whereas the inferior vena cava is accessed from the femoral vein. The insertion requires a minor surgical procedure: percutaneous vein cannulation with the introduction of a catheter. The catheter may be a single or multilumen. A long-line peripheral catheter can also be used to access the superior vena cava. The long-line catheter is inserted in a large vein (the basilic) and advanced through the subclavian to the superior vena cava. In some states, the peripherally inserted central catheters (PICC), are inserted by registered nurses.

Patients who need IV access for long-term use, such as chemotherapy, antibiotic therapy, or nutritional support, are given much longer catheters, which are tunneled under the skin after the vein is cannulated. The catheter and its drug infusion port exits from the subcutaneous tissue to a site on the chest. Examples of these devices are the Hickman, Groshong, and Cook.

Another type of catheter for long-term use has an implantable infusion port that is inserted in the subcutaneous tissue under the skin. These devices are called vascular access ports and they have a larger drug port or septum than other catheters. Care must be taken to use a noncoring needle that slices the port instead of making holes so that the septum will close instead of leak after the needle has been removed (Fig. 8–1).

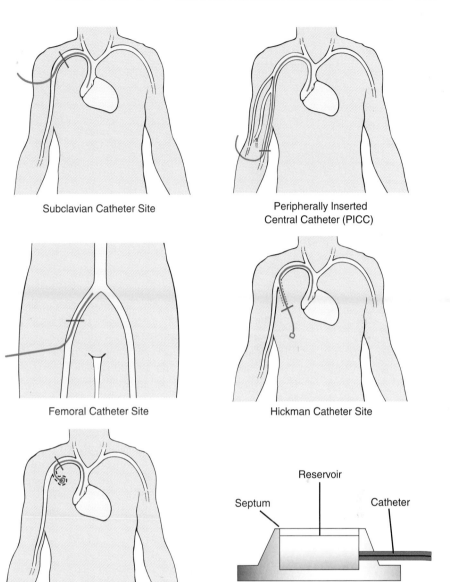

Subclavian Catheter Site

Peripherally Inserted
Central Catheter (PICC)

Femoral Catheter Site

Hickman Catheter Site

Subclavian Catheter
with Vascular Access Port

Vascular Access Port

FIGURE 8–1
Types of central venous access sites.

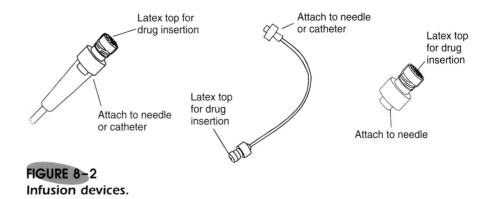

FIGURE 8-2
Infusion devices.

Intermittent Infusion Devices

When IV access sites are not used for continuous infusion but for intermittent therapy, they must be irrigated periodically to maintain patency. An intermittent infusion device can be attached to the end of the IV catheter or needle to close the connection that was attached to the IV tubing (Fig. 8–2). These devices have ports (stoppers) where needles or IV tubing can be inserted when drug therapy is resumed. This practice can eliminate the need for a constant low-rate infusion to keep the vein open (KVO) and reduce excessive fluid intake. The use of intermittent infusion devices can allow the patient more mobility and can be cost-effective because less IV tubing, IV solution, and regulating equipment are needed. To maintain patency of the IV sites, they can be irrigated either every 8 hours or before and after each drug infusion, depending on each institutions policy. Peripheral sites are irrigated or flushed with 1 to 3 mL of normal saline. Central venous sites are flushed with a heparinized saline solution. The amount of heparin used varies; 10 U/1 mL to 100 U/1 mL is the dosage range commonly given, but each institution's policies and procedures should be followed. The volume of the flush solution can vary with the type of venous access device and length of catheter tubing (Table 8–1).

TABLE 8-1
Venous Access Devices: Flushing Guidelines for Intermittent Use

TYPE	LENGTH (inches)	FLUSH SOLUTION	VOLUME (mL)	FREQUENCY
Peripheral	1–2	Normal saline	1–3	After each use or q8h
Central Venous				
Single-lumen	8	Heparinized saline	1	After each use or q8h
Multi-lumen	8	Heparinized saline	1/port	After each use or q8h
External-tunneled Hickman, Cook, or Groshong	35	Heparinized saline	2–5	After each use or q8h
Peripherally inserted central catheter	20	Normal saline	3–5	After each use or q12h
Implanted vascular access device	35	Heparinized saline	3–5	After each use; q5–7d when not in use

CONTINUOUS INTRAVENOUS ADMINISTRATION

When IV solutions are required, the physician orders the amount of solution per liter or milliliter to be administered for a time period, such as for 24 hours. The nurse calculates the IV flow rate according to the drop factor, the amount of fluids to be administered, and the time period.

Intravenous Sets

There are various IV infusion sets. The drop factor, or the number of drops per milliliter, is usually printed on the package. Sets that deliver large drops per milliliter (10–20 gtt/mL) are referred to as macrodrip sets, and those with small drops per milliliter (60 gtt/mL) are called microdrip or minidrip sets.

Examples of sets that deliver macrodrip (large drops) or microdrip (small drops) are listed in Table 8–2. Figures 8–3, 8–4, and 8–5 illustrate sizes of IV drops, IV bags and bottles, and IV tubing.

All microdrip sets deliver 60 gtt/mL. To determine the drop factor (gtt/mL), check the box or package of the IV set. This information is needed to calculate and regulate IV flow rate. In most instances, the nurse has a choice in using either the macrodrip or microdrip set. If the IV rate is to infuse at 100 mL/hour or faster, the macrodrip set is generally used. If the infusion rate is slower than 100 mL/hour, the microdrip is preferred. Slow drip rates of less than 100 mL/hour make macrodrip adjustment difficult. For example, at 50 mL/hour, the macrodrip rate would be 8 gtt/minute.

At times, IV fluids are given at a slow rate to *keep vein open* (KVO), also called *to keep open* (TKO). Reasons for ordering KVO include (1) a suspected or potential emergency situation requiring rapid administration of fluids and drugs and (2) maintaining an open line to give IV drugs at specified hours. For KVO, a microdrip set (60 gtt/mL) and a 250-mL IV bag can be used. KVO is usually regulated to deliver 10 mL/hour.

Calculation of Intravenous Flow Rate

Three different methods can be used to calculate IV flow rate (drops per minute or gtt/min). The nurse should select one of the methods, memorize it, and use it to calculate dosages.*

---

* The two-step method is the most commonly used method for calculating IV flow rate.

TABLE 8–2
Intravenous Sets

DROPS (gtt) PER MILLILITER	
Macrodrip sets 10 gtt/mL 15 gtt/mL 20 gtt/mL	Microdrip sets 60 gtt/mL

MACRODRIP AND MICRODRIP SIZES

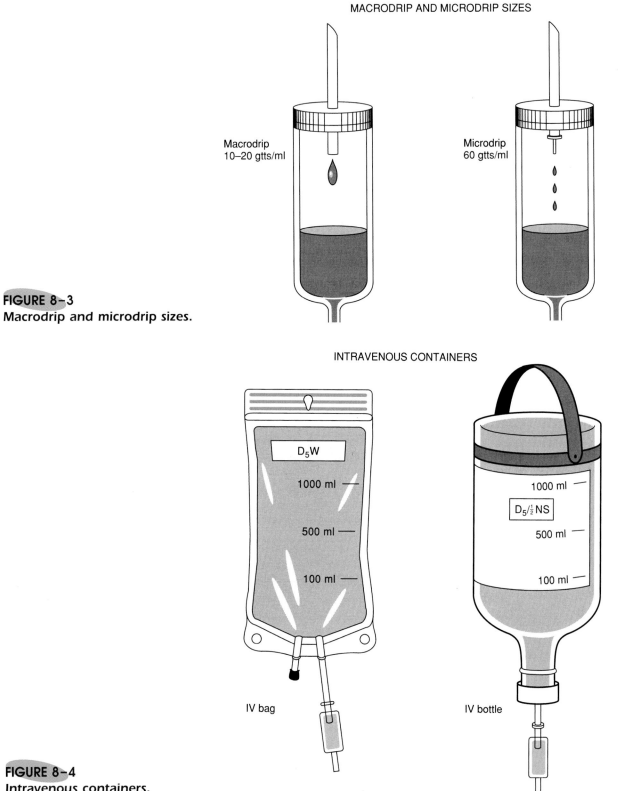

Macrodrip
10–20 gtts/ml

Microdrip
60 gtts/ml

FIGURE 8–3
Macrodrip and microdrip sizes.

INTRAVENOUS CONTAINERS

D₅W

1000 ml

500 ml

100 ml

D₅/½NS

1000 ml

500 ml

100 ml

IV bag

IV bottle

FIGURE 8–4
Intravenous containers.

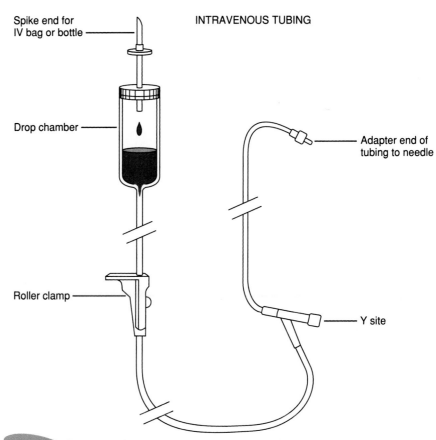

INTRAVENOUS TUBING

Spike end for
IV bag or bottle

Drop chamber

Adapter end of
tubing to needle

Roller clamp

Y site

FIGURE 8–5
Intravenous tubing.

Three-Step Method

a. $\dfrac{\text{amount of solution}}{\text{hours to administer}} = \text{mL/hr}$

b. $\dfrac{\text{mL per hour}}{60 \text{ minutes}} = \text{mL/min}$

c. mL per minute $\times$ gtt per mL of IV set = gtt/min

Two-Step Method

a. amount of fluid $\div$ hours to administer = mL/hr

b. $\dfrac{\text{mL per hour} \times \text{gtt/mL (IV set)}}{60 \text{ minutes}} = \text{gtt/min}$

One-Step Method

$$\dfrac{\text{amount fluid} \times \text{gtt/mL (IV set)}}{\text{hours to administer} \times \text{minutes per hour (60)}} = \text{gtt/min}$$

Safety Considerations

All IV infusions should be checked every hour to ensure the rate of infusion and to assess for potential problems. Common problems associated with IV infusions are kinked tubing, extravasation of IV fluids, and "runaway" IV rates. IVs using electronic IV delivery devices also need to be monitored. Mechanical problems or incorrect settings can cause incorrect fluid administration. Fluid overload, thrombus formation, and infiltration at the IV site are complications of IV therapy that can be avoided with frequent monitoring of the IV infusion. See Appendix A for more detailed information on safe nursing practice for IV drug administration.

Mixing Drugs Used for Continuous Intravenous Administration

Drugs such as multiple vitamins and potassium chloride can be added to the IV solution bag for continuous IV infusion. It is suggested that the drug or drugs be added to the bag or bottle immediately before administering the IV fluid. Inject the drug into the rubber stopper on the IV bag or bottle and rotate several times to ensure dispersal of the drug. Do *not* add the drug while the infusion is running unless the bag is rotated. A drug solution injected into an upright infusing IV solution causes the drug to concentrate into the lower portion of the IV bag and not be dispersed. The patient will receive a concentrated drug solution and this can be harmful (e.g., if the drug was potassium chloride). If drugs are injected into the IV bag prior to use, the bag should be refrigerated to maintain drug potency.

There are various nutrients (dextrose) and electrolytes in commercially prepared IV solutions. The commonly used solutions are dextrose in water, normal saline, one-half normal saline, and lactated Ringer's. These types of solutions are abbreviated as listed in Table 8–3.

EXAMPLES

Two problems for determining IV flow rate are given. Each problem is solved using each of the three methods for calculating IV flow rate.

PROBLEM 1: Order: 1000 mL of 5% D_5½ NSS (5% dextrose in ½ normal saline solution) in 6 hours.

TABLE 8–3
Abbreviations of Solutions

IV SOLUTION	ABBREVIATION
5% Dextrose in water	D_5W, 5% D/W
10% Dextrose in water	$D_{10}W$, 10% D/W
0.9% Sodium chloride, normal saline solution	0.9% NaCl, NSS, PSS
0.45% Sodium chloride, ½ normal saline solution	0.45% NaCl, ½ NSS, ½ PSS
5% Dextrose in 0.9% sodium chloride	D_5NSS, 5% D/NSS, 5% D/0.9% NaCl, D_5 PSS
5% Dextrose in 0.45% sodium chloride, 5% dextrose in ½ normal saline solution	D_5½ NSS, 5% D/½ NSS, ½ PSS
Lactated Ringer's solution	LRS

Available: 1 L (1000 mL) of $D_5\frac{1}{2}$ NSS solution bag; IV set labeled 10 gtt/mL.

How many drops per minute should the patient receive?

Three-Step Method: **a.** $\dfrac{1000 \text{ mL}}{6 \text{ hr}} = 166.6$ or 167 mL/hr

b. $\dfrac{167 \text{ mL}}{60 \text{ min}} = 2.7$ or 2.8 mL/min

c. 2.8 mL/min × 10 gtt/mL = 28 gtt/min

Two-Step Method: **a.** 1000 mL ÷ 6 hr = 167 mL/hr

b. $\dfrac{167 \text{ mL/hr} \times \overset{1}{\cancel{10}} \text{ gtt/mL}}{\underset{6}{\cancel{60}} \text{ min}} = \dfrac{167}{6} = 28$ gtt/min

10 and 60 cancel to 1 and 6.

If mL/hr is given, use only part **b** of the two-step method for calculating IV flow rate.

One-Step Method: $\dfrac{1000 \text{ mL} \times \overset{1}{\cancel{10}} \text{ gtt/mL}}{6 \text{ hr} \times \underset{6}{\cancel{60}} \text{ min}} \times \dfrac{1000}{36} = 27\text{--}28$ gtt/min

10 and 60 cancel to 1 and 6.

The use of a hand calculator is highly suggested to avoid errors.

Answer: 28 gtt/minute.

PROBLEM 2: Order: 1000 mL of D_5W (5% dextrose in water), 1 vial of MVI (multiple vitamin), and 20 mEq of KCl (potassium chloride) every 8 hours.

Available: 1000 mL D_5W solution bag
1 vial of MVI = 5 mL
40 mEq/20 mL of KCl in an ampule
IV set labeled 15 gtt/mL

How many milliliters of KCl would you withdraw as equivalent to 20 mEq of KCl?
How would you mix KCl in the IV bag?
How many drops per minute should the patient receive?

Procedure: MVI: inject 5 mL of MVI into the rubber stopper on the IV bag.
KCl: calculate the prescribed dosage for KCl using the basic formula or ratio and proportion.

$$\frac{D}{H} \times V = \frac{20}{40} \times 20 \quad \textbf{or}$$

$$= \frac{400}{40} = 10 \text{ mL}$$

H : V :: D : X
40 mEq : 20 mL : : 20 mEq : X mL

40 X = 400
X = 10 mL

Withdraw 10 mL of KCl and inject into the rubber stopper on the IV bag. Make sure the KCl solution is dispersed throughout the IV solution by rotating the IV bag.

Three-Step Method: **a.** $\dfrac{1000 \text{ mL}}{8 \text{ hr}} = 125 \text{ mL/hr}$

b. $\dfrac{125 \text{ mL}}{60 \text{ min}} = 2.0\text{–}2.1 \text{ mL/min}$

c. $2.1 \times 15 = 31\text{–}32 \text{ gtt/min}$

Two-Step Method: **a.** $1000 \div 8 = 125 \text{ mL/hr}$

b. $\dfrac{125 \text{ mL/hr} \times \overset{1}{\cancel{15}} \text{ gtt/mL}}{\underset{4}{\cancel{60}} \text{ min}} = \dfrac{125}{4} = 31\text{–}32 \text{ gtt/min}$

15 and 60 cancel to 1 and 4.

IV flow rate should be 31 to 32 gtt/min.

One-Step Method: $\dfrac{1000 \text{ mL} \times \overset{1}{\cancel{15}} \text{ gtt/mL}}{8 \text{ hr} \times \underset{4}{\cancel{60}} \text{ min}} = \dfrac{1000}{32} = 32 \text{ gtt/min}$

15 and 60 cancel to 1 and 4.

IV flow rate should be 31 to 32 gtt/min.

Note:

Medication volume can be added to the total volume if strict intake and output is being recorded. In general, an IV bag contains more fluid than labeled on the bag; some estimates are as much as 50 mL. If an electric infusion device is used, the patient will get the amount programed in the device. When the volume of the medication exceeds 20 mL, the amount should be added to the total volume to be infused. If the volume is less than 20 mL, it will not greatly change the hourly rate.

I. Practice Problems: Continuous Intravenous Administration

Select *one* of the three methods for calculating IV flow rate. The two-step method is preferred by most nurses.

1. Order: 1000 mL of D_5W to run for 12 hours.
   a. Would you use a macrodrip or microdrip IV set? _____
   b. Calculate the drops per minute (gtt/min) using one of the three methods. _____

2. Order: 3 L of IV solutions for 24 hours: 2 L of 5% D/½ NSS and 1 L of D_5W.
   a. One liter is equal to _____ mL.

    b. Each liter should run for _____ hours.

    c. The institution uses an IV set with a drop factor of 15 gtt/mL. How many drops per minute should the patient receive? _____

3. Order: 250 mL of D_5W for KVO.

    a. What type of IV set would you use? _____
    Why? _____

    b. How many drops per minute should the patient receive? _____

4. Order: 1000 mL of 5% D/0.2% NaCl with 10 mEq of KCl for 10 hours. Available: macrodrip IV set with a drop factor of 20 gtt/mL and microdrip set; KCl 20 mEq/20 mL vial.

    a. How many milliliters of KCl should be injected into the IV bag? _
    _____

    b. How is KCl mixed in the IV solution? _____

    c. How many drops per minute should the patient receive using the macrodrip set and the microdrip set? _____

5. A liter (1000 mL) of IV fluid was started at 9 AM and was to run for 8 hours. The IV set delivers 15 gtt/mL. Four hours later, only 300 mL have been absorbed.

    a. How much IV fluid is left? _____

    b. Recalculate the flow rate for the remaining IV fluids. _____

6. The patient is to receive 100 mL/hr of D_5W.
    Available: Microdrip set (60 gtt/mL.)
    How many drops per minute should the patient receive? _____

INTERMITTENT INTRAVENOUS ADMINISTRATION

There are many advantages of giving drugs via the intermittent IV route. The IV route allows for rapid therapeutic concentration of the drug and control over the onset of action and peak concentrations. Blood serum concentrations can be achieved via the IV route if the oral route is unavailable because of the patient's condition, such as gastrointestinal malabsorption or neurologic deficits that prevent swallowing. The IV route can be used on an outpatient basis and can ensure compliance with drug therapy. The IV route also allows for the rapid correction of electrolyte imbalances. IV medications can be given at intervals within a 24-hour period for days or weeks. These medications are administered in a small volume of fluid (50 to 250 mL of D_5W or saline). The drug solution is usually delivered to the patient in 15 minutes to 1 hour, depending on the medication. A separate delivery set or secondary set is used for intermittent therapy if the patient is also receiving continuous infusion through the same IV site.

Secondary Intravenous Sets Without Controllers

Two sets available for administering IV drugs are (1) the calibrated cylinder (chamber) with tubing, such as Buretrol, Volutrol, and Soluset; and (2) the second-

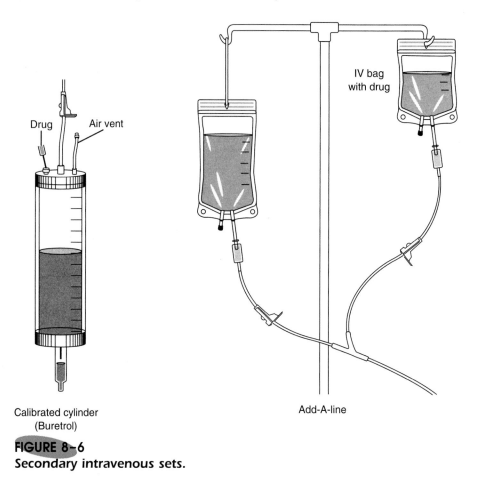

Drug   Air vent

Calibrated cylinder
(Buretrol)

IV bag
with drug

Add-A-line

FIGURE 8–6
Secondary intravenous sets.

ary set, which is similar to a regular IV set except that the tubing is shorter (Fig. 8–6). The secondary set is primarily used for infusing small volumes, such as 50-, 100-, and 250-mL bags or bottles. The chambers of the Buretrol, Volutrol, and Soluset devices each hold 150 mL of solution. Medication is injected into the chamber and diluted with solution. These methods for administering IV drugs are referred to as IV piggyback (IVPB). Usually, drugs administered by Buretrol, Volutrol, or Soluset are prepared by the nurse.

Normally, drugs for IV infusion are diluted prior to infusion. Clinical agencies frequently have their own protocols for dilutions; if not, the drug circular should have infusion guidelines. if the information is not available, the hospital pharmacy should be contacted. Guidelines and protocols help in preventing drug and fluid incompatibility.

NOTE:

When using Buretrol, 15 mL of IV solution should be added to flush the drug out of the IV line after the drug infusion is completed. Flush volume is added to patient intake.

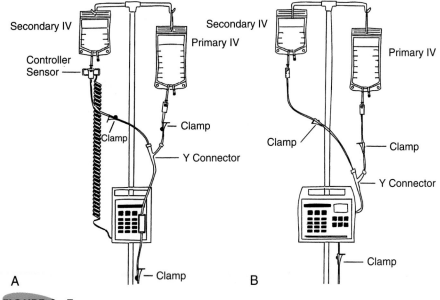

FIGURE 8–7
(A) **Volumetric infusion controller.** *(B)* **Volumetric infusion pump.**

Electronic Intravenous Delivery Devices

Controllers and pumps are the two basic types of electronic IV delivery devices. Controllers (Fig. 8–7A) work by the pressure that gravity exerts on the fluid in the IV container, bag, or bottle. They have an electronically controlled clamp that adjusts the flow by clamping and releasing the IV tubing. The controller's drop sensor on the drip chamber detects any increase or decrease of drops and automatically adjusts the clamp. Controllers are sensitive to any restrictions, such as infiltrations, and an alarm is sounded when the set rate cannot be maintained. Controllers are not accurate for volumes less than 5 mL/hr. To ensure the correct rate of infusion, the IV bag or bottle must be three feet above the IV site, and the tubing must be free of occlusions.

There are two types of pumps; the IV delivery pump (Fig. 8–7B) and the syringe pump. The IV pump will work on gravity but exerts positive pressure if there is any resistance. Pumps do not recognize infiltrations. The alarm will not sound until the pump has exerted its maximum pressure to overcome resistance. Syringe pumps are primarily used when a small volume of medication is given. Some syringe pumps can operate with syringes of various sizes, from tuberculin to 35 mL. Syringe pumps are primarily used in neonatal and critical care units.

IV pumps are recommended for use with all central venous lines, arterial lines, and hyperalimentation. Controllers are used for peripheral lines, especially if fluid overload is a concern, or for the need to decrease the risk of infiltration with irritating drugs such as potassium chloride. A combination controller/pump delivery device is used as an infusion controller, as an infusion pump, or both (Fig. 8–8). This volumetric infusion pump/controller can simultaneously infuse two solutions in the same site or in independent sites, at the same or different rates. It can function as two pumps, as two controllers, or as a pump and a controller.

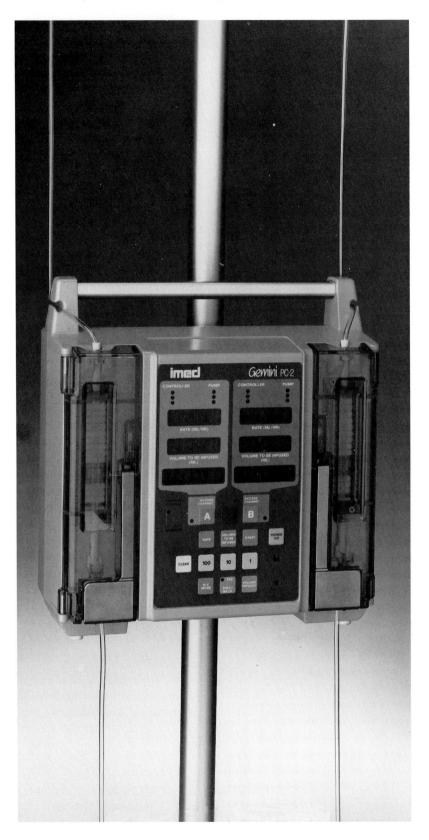

FIGURE 8–8
IMED Gemini PC2 Volumetric Infusion Pump/controller regulator. (Courtesy of IMED Corporation, San Diego, CA.)

Another type of delivery device that is inexpensive is the Dial-A-Flow. The dial on the tubing is turned to the desired rate of IV flow per hour (mL/hr). Dial-A-Flow is primarily used for controlling large volumes of IV solutions and for preventing runaway IV flow and variations in the IV flow rate.

Flow Rates for Regulators

Determining the flow rates for electronic delivery devices depends on whether the type of flow control is volumetric or nonvolumetric. Volumetric delivery devices deliver a specific volume of fluid at a specific rate, measured in milliliters per hour (mL/hr). Nonvolumetric delivery devices are designed to infuse at a drop rate (gtt/min). Distinguishing between volumetric and nonvolumetric delivery devices involves checking the calibration on the machine display for rate units (mL/hr or gtt/min).

Calculating Flow Rates for Intravenous Drugs and Electrolytes

Drugs that are given by intermittent infusion must be diluted and infused slowly. The pH and the osmolality determine the dilution. A slower infusion time allows for the medication to be diluted in the blood vessel, which can prevent phlebitis and high concentrations of drug in plasma and tissues causing time-related overdose, toxicity, or allergic reaction. Drug-dosing instructions indicate the amount and type of solution and the length of infusion time. The nurse must calculate the drug dose from the physician's order, then calculate the flow rate from the drug-dosing information.

When calibrated cylinders, Volutrol, Buretrol, or Soluset, are used for drug infusion, the tubing must be flushed after each infusion to make sure the entire drug dose was given. The rinse can range from 10 to 25 mL and is added to the IV intake. When a minibag is used, the IV tubing should be drained so the patient receives the complete dose.

1. Secondary sets (calibrated cylinders and 50- to 250-mL IV bags) use drops per minute (gtt/min). The one-step method for calculating drops per minute (gtt/min) is used when administering IV drugs by secondary sets.

One-Step Method for IV Drug Calculation with Secondary Set

$$\frac{\text{amount of solution} \times \text{gtt/mL of the set}}{\text{minutes to administer}} = \text{gtt/min}$$

2. Volumetric regulators use units of milliliters per hour. Use the following method to calculate milliliters per hour.

$$\text{Amount of solution} \div \frac{\text{minutes to administer}}{\text{60 minutes/hour}} = \text{mL/hr}$$

NOTE:

Medication volume should be added to the dilution volume in intermittent drug therapy if the volume exceeds 5 mL. Because smaller volumes of fluid are used for IV infusion, drug dosage may be decreased if the volume of medication is not included in the dilution volume. The amount of solution in the formula should include both volumes.

EXAMPLES

PROBLEM 1: Order: Tagamet 200 mg, IV, q6h.
Drug available: cimetidine (Tagamet) 300 mg/2 mL vial in aqueous solution.
Set and solution: Buretrol set with drop factor of 60 gtt/mL; 500 mL of D$_5$W.
Instruction: Dilute drug in 100 mL of D$_5$W and infuse over 20 minutes.

Drug Calculation:

$$\frac{D}{H} \times V = \frac{200}{300} \times 2 \quad \textbf{or}$$

$$= \frac{400}{300}$$

X = 1.3 mL of Tagamet

H   :   V   ::   D   :   X
300 mg : 2 mL :: 200 mg : X mL

300 X = 400

$$X = \frac{400}{300} = 300\overline{)400.0}^{\,1.3}$$

X = 1.3 mL of Tagamet

Flow Rate Calculation:

$$\frac{\text{amount of solution} \times \text{gtt/mL}}{\text{minutes to administer}} = \frac{100 \text{ mL} \times \overset{3}{\cancel{60}} \text{ gtt}}{\underset{1}{\cancel{20}}} = 300 \text{ gtt/min}$$

Answer: Inject 1.3 mL of Tagamet into 100 mL of D$_5$W in the Buretrol chamber.
Regulate IV flow rate to 300 gtt/min.
It would be impossible to count 300 gtt/min. Instead of using the Buretrol, the nurse could use a secondary set with a larger drop factor or a regulator. If the Buretrol is the only available secondary IV set, then the 300 gtt/min rate should be approximated.

PROBLEM 2: Order: Mandol 500 mg, IV, q6h.
Drug available: cefamandole (Mandol) 2 g vial in powdered form. Add 6.6 mL of diluent = 8 mL of drug solution (2g = 8 mL).

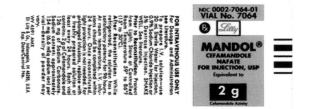

Set and solution: secondary set with 100 mL D$_5$W and a drop factor of 15 gtt/mL.
Instruction: dilute in 100 mL of D$_5$W and infuse over 30 minutes.

Drug Calculation: (2.0 g = 2.000 mg)

$$\frac{D}{H} \times V = \frac{500}{2000} \times 8 \qquad \text{or} \qquad \begin{array}{ccccccc} H & : & V & : : & D & : & X \\ 2000 \text{ mg} & : & 8 \text{ mL} & : : & 500 \text{ mg} & : & X \text{ mL} \end{array}$$

$$= \frac{4000}{2000} = 2 \text{ mL of Mandol} \qquad\qquad \begin{array}{c} 2000 \text{ X} = 4000 \\ \text{X} = 2 \text{ mL of Mandol} \end{array}$$

Flow Rate Calculation:

$$\frac{\text{amount of solution} \times \text{gtt/mL}}{\text{minutes to administer}} = \frac{100 \text{ mL} \times \overset{1}{\cancel{15}}}{\underset{2}{\cancel{30}}} = \frac{100}{2} = 50 \text{ gtt/min}$$

Answer: Inject 2 mL of Mandol into the 100 mL D_5W bag. Regulate IV flow rate at 50 gtt/min.

PROBLEM 3: Order: ampicillin (Polycillin-N) 1 g, IV, q6h.
Drug available:

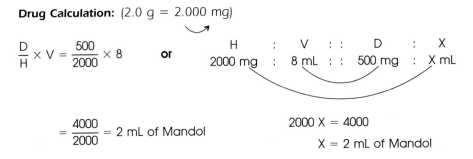

Add 4.5 mL of diluent, which equals 5 mL.
Set: use a volumetric pump.
Instruction: dilute in 50 mL of D_5W and infuse over 15 minutes.

Drug Calculation: ampicillin 1 g = 5 mL of drug solution.

Volumetric Pump Rate: amount of solution ÷ $\dfrac{\text{minutes to administer}}{60 \text{ minutes}}$ = mL/hr

$$55 \text{ mL} \div \frac{15 \text{ min}}{60 \text{ min}} = 55 \times \frac{\overset{4}{\cancel{60}}}{\underset{1}{\cancel{15}}} = 220 \text{ mL/hr}$$

Note: Amount of solution is 50 mL of D_5W + 5 mL medication = 55 mL.

Answer: Rate on volumetric pump should be set at 220 mL/hr to deliver ampicillin 1 g in 15 minutes.

PROBLEM 4: Order: albumin 25 g, IV.
Available: albumin 25 g in 50 mL.
Set: use a volumetric pump.
Instruction: administer over 25 minutes, or 2 mL/min.

Drug Calculation: Not applicable.

Volumetric Pump Rate:

$$50 \text{ mL} \div \frac{25 \text{ min}}{60 \text{ min}} = 50 \times \frac{60}{25} = \frac{3000}{25} = 120 \text{ mL/hr}$$

Answer: Volumetric rate should be set at 120 mL/hr.

PROBLEM 5: Order: potassium phosphate 10 mM IV in 100 mL NSS over 90 minutes.
Drug available:

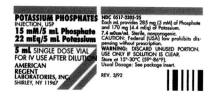

Set: use volumetric pump.

Drug Calculation:

$$\frac{D}{H} \times V = \frac{10}{15} \times 5 \quad \textbf{or}$$

$$= \frac{50}{15}$$

$$= 3.3 \text{ mL of potassium phosphate}$$

H	:	V	: :	D	:	V
15 mm	:	5 mL	: :	10 mm	:	X mL

$$15 \text{ X} = 50$$
$$\text{X} = 3.3 \text{ mL of potassium phosphate}$$

Volumetric Pump Rate:

$$\text{amount of solution} \div \frac{\text{minutes to administer}}{60 \text{ minutes}} = \text{mL/hr}$$

$$100 \text{ mL} \div \frac{90 \text{ min}}{60 \text{ min}} = 100 \times \frac{60}{90} = 66.6 \text{ or } 67 \text{ mL/hr}$$

Answer: Rate on the volumetric pump should be 67 mL/hr to deliver potassium phosphate 10 mM in 90 minutes.

NOTE:

When administering the electrolyte potassium, the maximum infusion rate is 10 mEq/hr.

II. Practice Problems: Intermittent Intravenous Administration

Calculate the fluid rate by using a calibrated cylinder (Buretrol), secondary set, or a volumetric pump, as indicated in each question.

1. Order: cephapirin (Cefadyl) 500 mg, IV, q6h.
Drug available:

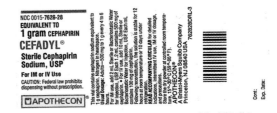

Drug label: add _____ mL of diluent _____;
1 g = _____ mL; 100 mg = 1 mL. What type of syringe should be used? _____
Set and solution: Buretrol set with a drop factor of 60 gtt/mL; 500 mL of D_5W.
Instruction: dilute drug in 75 mL of D_5W and infuse over 30 minutes.

Drug calculation:

_____

Flow rate calculation:

_____

2. Order: oxacillin (Prostaphlin) 400 mg, IV, q6h.
Drug available:

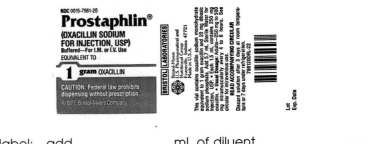

Drug label: add _____ mL of diluent _____ ;
250 mg = _____ mL; 1 g = _____ mL.
Set and solution: secondary set with a drop factor of 15 gtt/mL; 500 mL of D_5W.
Instruction: dilute drug in 100 mL of D_5W and infuse over 40 minutes.

Drug calculation:

_____

Flow rate calculation:

_____

3. Order: nafcillin (Nafcil) 1 g, IV, q6h.
Drug available:

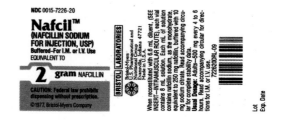

Set and solution: Buretrol set with a drop factor of 60 gtt/mL;
volumetric pump; 500 mL of D_5W.
Instruction: dilute drug in 75 mL of D_5W and infuse over 40 minutes.

Drug calculation:

_____

Flow rate calculation (gtt/min):
How many drops per minute should the patient receive using the Buretrol set?

_____

Volumetric pump rate (mL/hr):
With a volumetric pump, how many mL/hr should be administered?

_____

4. Order: piperacillin 2.5 g, IV, q6h.
Drug available: piperacillin 4 g vial in powdered form; add 7.8 mL of diluent to yield 10 mL of drug solution (4 g = 10 mL).
Set and solution: Buretrol set with a drop factor of 60 gtt/mL;
volumetric pump; 500 mL of D_5W.
Instruction: dilute drug in 100 mL of D_5W and infuse over 30 minutes.

Drug calculation:

_____

Flow rate calculation (gtt/min):
How many drops per minute should the patient receive using the Buretrol set?

_____

Volumetric pump rate (mL/hr):
With a volumetric pump, how many mL/hr should be administered?

_____

5. Order: methicillin (Staphcillin) 1 g, IV, q6h.
Drug available: Staphcillin 4 g in powdered form in vial; add 5.7 mL of diluent to yield 8 mL.

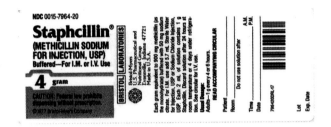

Set and solution: secondary set with a drop factor of 15 gtt/mL; 100 mL bag of D₅W; volumetric pump.
Instruction: dilute drug in 100 mL of D₅W and infuse over 40 minutes.

Drug calculation:

_____

Explain the procedure for diluting the drug and adding it to the IV bag.

_____

Flow rate calculation (gtt/min):
How many drops per minute should the patient receive using a secondary set?

_____

Volumetric pump rate (mL/hr):
With a volumetric pump, how many mL/hr should be administered?

_____

6. Order: Vibramycin 100 mg, IV, q12h.
Drug available: doxycycline (Vibramycin) 100-mg vial in powdered form; add 10 mL of diluent.

Set and solution: secondary set with a drop factor of 15 gtt/mL; 100 mL of D₅W; volumetric pump.
Instruction: dilute 10 mL in 90 mL of D₅W and infuse over 60 minutes.
Dilution should be 1 mg = 1 mL.

Drug calculation:

_____

Flow rate calculation (gtt/min):
How many drops per minute should the patient receive using the Buretrol set?

_____

Volumetric pump rate (mL/hr):
With a volumetric pump, how many mL/hr should be administered?

_____

7. Order: potassium chloride 20 mEq in 150 mL D_5W infused over 2 hours.
Drug available: KCl 40 mEq/20 mL

Set and solution: secondary set with drop factor 15 gtt/mL; 150 mL bottle D_5W; volumetric pump.

Drug calculation:

_____

Volumetric pump rate (mL/hr):
How many mL/hr should be administered?

_____

8. Order: magnesium sulfate 5 g in 100 mL D_5W infused over 3 hours.
Drug available: $MgSO_4$ 3 g/5 mL

Set and solution: secondary set with drip factor of 15 gtt/mL; 10 mL bag D_5W; volumetric pump.

Drug calculation:

_____

Volumetric pump rate (mL/hr):
How many mL/hr should be administered?

9. Order: calcium gluconate 10%, 16 mEq in 100 mL D_5W infused over 30 minutes.
Drug available:

CALCIUM GLUCONATE
INJECTION, USP
10%
23.25 mEq/50 mL Calcium
(0.465mEq/mL)

FOR SLOW
INTRAVENOUS USE
50mL
SINGLE DOSE VIAL
AMERICAN
REGENT
LABORATORIES, INC.
SUBSIDIARY OF
LUITPOLD PHARMACEUTICALS
SHIRLEY, NY 11967   REV. 1/91

NDC 0517-3950-25
Each mL contains: Calcium Gluconate
(Monohydrate) 98mg, Calcium Saccharate
(Tetrahydrate) 4.6mg, Water for Injection
q.s. pH adjusted with Sodium Hydroxide
and/or Hydrochloric Acid. Calcium Saccharate
provides 6.2% of the total Calcium content.
0.68mOsmol/mL Sterile, nonpyrogenic.
CAUTION: Federal Law (USA) Prohibits
Dispensing Without Prescription.
WARNING: DISCARD UNUSED PORTION
IF CRYSTALLIZATION OCCURS, WARMING
MAY DISSOLVE THE PRECIPITATE (See
Insert). THE INJECTION MUST BE CLEAR
AT THE TIME OF USE.
Directions for Use: See Insert

Set and solution: secondary set with a drip factor of 15 gtt/mL; 100 mL bag D_5W; volumetric pump.

Drug calculation:

_____

Volumetric pump rate (mL/hr):
How many mL/hr should be administered?

10. Order: potassium phosphate 6 mM and potassium chloride 40 mEq in 250 mL normal saline: infused over 6 hours.
Drug available: KCl 40 mEq/20 mL and

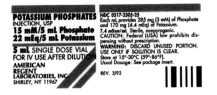

Set and solution: secondary set with a drip factor 15 gtt/mL; 250 mL NSS; volumetric pump.

Drug calculation:

_____

Volumetric pump rate (mL/hr):
How many mL/hr should be administered?

_____

When administering the electrolyte potassium, the maximum infusion rate is 10 mEq/hr. What is the total dosage of potassium in this order? Does it exceed 10 mEq/hr?

_____

ANSWERS

I. Continuous Intravenous Administration

1. a. Microdrip set, because the patient is to receive 83 mL/hr

b. Three-step method: (a) $\dfrac{1000}{12} = 83$ mL/hr   (b) $\dfrac{83}{60} = 1.38$ mL/min

(c) 1.4 mL/min $\times$ 60 gtt/mL = 84 gtt/min

Using a microdrip set (60 gtt/mL), IV should run 84 gtt/min.

2. a. 1 L = 1000 mL
b. Each liter should run for 8 hours.
c. Two-step method: 1000 ÷ 8 = 125 mL/hr

$$\frac{125 \times \cancel{15}^{\,1}}{\underset{4}{\cancel{60}}} = \frac{125}{4} = 31\text{–}32 \text{ gtt/min}$$

Using a 15 gtt/mL drop set, IV should run 31–32 gtt/min.

3. a. Microdrip set with drop factor of 60 gtt/mL

b. One-step method: $\dfrac{250 \times \overset{1}{\cancel{60}}}{24 \times \underset{1}{\cancel{60}}} = 10$ gtt/min

Using a microdrip set, IV should run 10 gtt/min. KVO usually means 24 hours.

4. a. 10 mL of KCl
   b. Use a 10-mL syringe, withdraw 10 mL of KCl and inject into the rubber port stopper of the IV bag.
   c. Microdrip set: 100 gtt/min
      Macrodrip set: drop factor of 20 gtt/mL; 34 gtt/min

5. a. 700 mL of IV fluid is left and 4 hours are left.
   b. Recalculate using 700 mL and 4 hours to run.

   Three-step method: (a) $\dfrac{700}{4} = 175$ mL/hr

   (b) $\dfrac{175}{60} = 2.9$ mL/min

   (c) $2.9 \times 15 = 44$ gtt/min

6. 100 gtt/min

   Two-step method: $\dfrac{100 \times \overset{1}{\cancel{60}} \text{ gtt/mL}}{\underset{1}{\cancel{60}} \text{ min}} = 100$ gtt/min

II. Intermittent Intravenous Administration

1. Add 10 mL of sterile or bacteriostatic water (1 g = 10 mL).
   Drug calculation: change 500 mg to grams because the drug label is in grams. Move the decimal point three spaces to the *left:* 500. mg = 0.5 g.

   $\dfrac{D}{H} \times V = \dfrac{0.5}{1} \times 10$ mL   **or**   H : V : : D : X
                                                1 g : 10 mL : : 0.5 g : X mL

   $= \dfrac{5}{1} = 5$ mL Cefadyl $1 X = 10 \times 0.5$

                           $X = 5$ mL Cefadyl

   Use a 10-mL syringe to reconstitute the drug.
   Flow rate calculation:

   $\dfrac{\text{amount of solution} \times \text{gtt/mL (set)}}{\text{minutes to administer}} = \dfrac{75 \text{ mL} \times \overset{2}{\cancel{60}} \text{ gtt/mL}}{\underset{1}{\cancel{30}} \text{ minutes}} = 150$ gtt/min

   Regulate flow rate for 150 gtt/min.

2. Add 5.7 mL of sterile water.
   250 mg = 1.5 mL; 1 g = 6 mL (250 mg is ¼ of a gram; 4 × 1.5 = 6 mL)

   Drug calculation: change 400 mg to grams because the drug label is in grams. Move the decimal point three spaces to the *left:* 400. mg = 0.4 g.

$$\frac{0.4}{1} \times 6 \text{ mL} = 2.4 \text{ mL of Prostaphlin} \quad \textbf{or} \quad 1 \text{ g} : 6 \text{ mL} :: 0.4 \text{ g} : X \text{ mL}$$

$$1 X = 6 \times 0.4$$
$$X = 2.4 \text{ mL of}$$
$$\text{Prostaphlin}$$

Flow rate calculation:

$$\frac{100 \text{ mL} \times 15 \text{ gtt/mL (set)}}{40 \text{ minutes}} = 37.5 \text{ or } 38 \text{ gtt/min}$$

Regulate flow rate for 38 gtt/min.

3. *Drug calculation:* Nafcillin 2 g = 8 mL; 1 g = 4 mL
   Flow rate calculation: total solution: 75 mL D_5W + 4 mL of drug solution = 79 mL
   Buretrol set:

$$\frac{79 \text{ mL} \times \overset{3}{\cancel{60}} \text{ gtt/mL (set)}}{\underset{2}{\cancel{40}} \text{ minutes}} = \frac{237}{2} = 118.5 \text{ or } 119 \text{ gtt/min}$$

Volumetric pump set:

$$\text{amount of solution} \div \frac{\text{minutes to administer}}{60 \text{ min/hr}} = \text{mL/hr}$$

$$79 \text{ mL} \div \frac{\overset{2}{\cancel{40}} \text{ min to administer}}{\underset{3}{\cancel{60}} \text{ min/hr}} = 79 \times \frac{3}{2} = \frac{237}{2} = 119 \text{ mL/hr}$$

Set volumetric rate at 119 mL/hr to deliver Nafcillin 1 g in 40 minutes.

4. *Drug calculation:*

$$\frac{D}{H} \times V = \frac{2.5 \text{ g}}{\underset{2}{\cancel{4} \text{ g}}} \times \overset{5}{\cancel{10}} \text{ mL} \quad \textbf{or} \quad H : V :: D : X$$
$$\qquad\qquad\qquad\qquad\qquad 4 \text{ g} : 10 \text{ mL} :: 2.5 \text{ g} : X \text{ mL}$$

$$= \frac{12.5}{2} = 6.25 \text{ mL} \qquad\qquad 4 X = 25$$
$$\qquad\qquad\qquad\qquad\qquad\qquad X = 6.25 \text{ mL}$$

piperacillin 2.5 g = 6.25 mL

Flow rate calculation:
Buretrol set:

$$\frac{100 \text{ mL} \times \overset{2}{\cancel{60}} \text{ gtt/mL}}{\underset{1}{\cancel{30}} \text{ min/hr}} = 200 \text{ gtt/minute}$$

Volumetric pump rate: 100 mL + 6 mL medication = 106 mL

$$106 \text{ mL} \div \frac{\overset{1}{\cancel{30}} \text{ min to administer}}{\underset{2}{\cancel{60}} \text{ min/hr}} = 106 \times \frac{2}{1} = 212 \text{ mL/hr}$$

Set volumetric rate at 212 mL/hr to deliver piperacillin 2.5 g in 30 minutes.

5. *Drug calculation:*
   Staphcillin 4 g = 8 mL. Withdraw 2 mL from vial to yield Staphcillin 1 g.

Flow rate calculation:
Secondary set:

$$\frac{\overset{5}{\cancel{100}} \text{ mL} \times 15 \text{ gtt/mL (set)}}{\underset{2}{\cancel{40}} \text{ minutes}} = \frac{75}{2} = 37.5 \text{ or } 38 \text{ gtt/min}$$

Volumetric pump set:

$$100 \text{ mL} \times \frac{\overset{2}{\cancel{40}} \text{ min to administer}}{\underset{3}{\cancel{60}} \text{ min/hr}} = 100 \times \frac{3}{2} = \frac{300}{2} = 150 \text{ mL/hr}$$

Set volumetric rate at 150 mL/hr to deliver Staphcillin 1 g in 40 minutes.

6. *Drug calculation:* Mix 10 mL of diluent with Vibramycin 100 mg in vial.
Flow rate calculation: Expel 10 mL of IV solution. Inject 10 mL of drug solution into 90 mL of IV solution.

Secondary set:

$$\frac{100 \text{ mL} \times \overset{1}{\cancel{15}} \text{ gtt/mL}}{\underset{4}{\cancel{60}} \text{ minutes}} = \frac{100}{4} = 25 \text{ gtt/min}$$

Volumetric pump set:

$$100 \text{ mL} \div \frac{\overset{1}{\cancel{60}} \text{ minutes to administer}}{\underset{1}{\cancel{60}} \text{ min/hr}} = 100 \text{ mL/hr}$$

Set volumetric rate at 100 mL/hr to deliver Vibramycin 100 mg in 60 minutes.

7. *Drug calculation:*

$$\frac{D}{H} \times V = \frac{20}{40} \times 20 \quad \textbf{or} \qquad H \quad : \quad V \quad :: \quad D \quad : \quad X$$
$$\qquad\qquad\qquad\qquad\qquad\qquad\qquad 40 \quad : \quad 20 \quad :: \quad 20 \quad : \quad X$$
$$= \frac{400}{40} \qquad\qquad\qquad\qquad\qquad 40 \, X = 400$$
$$= 10 \text{ mL KCl} \qquad\qquad\qquad\quad X = 10 \text{ mL KCl}$$

Amount of solution: 150 mL + 10 mL = 160 mL

Volumetric pump rate:

$$160 \text{ mL} \div \frac{120 \text{ min to administer}}{60 \text{ min/hr}} = 160 \times \frac{1}{2} = 80 \text{ mL/hr}$$

Set volumetric pump rate at 80 mL/hr to deliver KCl 20 mEq in 2 hr.

8. *Drug Calculation:*

$$\frac{D}{H} \times V = \frac{5}{3} \times 5 \quad \textbf{or} \qquad H \quad : \quad V \quad :: \quad D \quad : \quad X$$
$$\qquad\qquad\qquad\qquad\qquad\qquad\qquad 3 \quad : \quad 5 \quad :: \quad 5 \quad : \quad X$$
$$= \frac{25}{3} \qquad\qquad\qquad\qquad\qquad 3 \, X = 25$$
$$= 8.3 \text{ mL MgSO}_4 \qquad\qquad\quad X = 8.3 \text{ mL MgSO}_4$$

Amount of solution: 8.3 mL + 100 mL = 108.3 mL

Volumetric pump rate:

$$108.3 \text{ mL} - \frac{180 \text{ min to administer}}{60 \text{ min/hr}} = 108.3 \times \frac{1}{3} = 36.1 \text{ mL/hr}$$

Set volumetric pump rate at 36 mL/hr to deliver $MgSO_4$ 5 g in 3 hr.

9. *Drug Calculation:*

$$\frac{D}{H} \times V = \frac{16}{23.25} \times 50 \quad \textbf{or} \qquad \begin{array}{ccccccc} H & : & V & :: & D & : & X \\ 23.25 & : & 50 & :: & 16 & : & X \end{array}$$

$$= \frac{800}{23.25} \qquad\qquad\qquad 23.25 \text{ X} = 800$$

$$\qquad\qquad\qquad\qquad\qquad X = 34.4 \text{ mL calcium}$$
$$\qquad\qquad\qquad\qquad\qquad\qquad\qquad \text{gluconate}$$

$$= 34.4 \text{ mL calcium gluconate}$$

Amount of solution: 34.4 mL + 100 mL = 134.4 mL

Volumetric pump rate:

$$134.4 \text{ mL} - \frac{30 \text{ min to administer}}{60 \text{ min/hr}} = 134.4 \times \frac{2}{1} = 268.8 \text{ or } 269 \text{ mL/hr}$$

10. *Drug Calculation:*

$$\frac{D}{H} \times V = \frac{6}{15} \times 5 \quad \textbf{or} \qquad \begin{array}{ccccccc} H & : & V & :: & D & : & X \\ 15 \text{ mm} & : & 5 & :: & 6 \text{ mm} & : & X \end{array}$$

$$= \frac{30}{15} \qquad\qquad\qquad 15 \text{ X} = 30$$

$$\qquad\qquad\qquad\qquad\qquad X = 2 \text{ mL } KPO_4$$

$$= 2 \text{ mL } KPO_4$$

KPO_4 2 mL + KCl 20 mL = 22 mL   22 mL + 250 mL = 272 mL

$$272 \text{ mL} - \frac{360 \text{ min to administer}}{60 \text{ min/hr}} = 272 \times \frac{1}{6} = 45.3 \text{ mL/hr}$$

Set volumetric rate at 45 mL/hr to deliver KPO_4 6 mM and KCl 40 mEq in 6 hr.

Amount of K in 6 mm potassium phosphate:

$$\begin{array}{ccccccc} 22 \text{ meq} & : & 5 \text{ mL} & :: & X & : & 2 \text{ mL} \end{array}$$
$$5 \text{ X} = 44$$
$$X = 8.8 \text{ mEq or } 9 \text{ mEq K/2mL of } KPO_4$$

KCl 40 mEq + 9 mEq K = 49 mEq in total dose over 6 hours
Does *not* exceed 10 mEq/m.

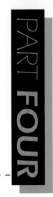

PART FOUR

Calculations for Specialty Areas

Pediatrics

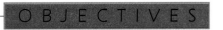

OBJECTIVES

- Utilize the two primary methods in determining pediatric drug dosages.
- State the reason for checking pediatric dosages prior to administration.
- Describe the dosage inaccuracies that can occur with pediatric drug formulas.
- Identify the steps in determining body surface area from a pediatric nomogram.

FACTORS INFLUENCING PEDIATRIC DRUG ADMINISTRATION

Drug dosages for children differ greatly from those for adults because of the physiologic differences between the two. Neonates and infants have immature kidney and liver function, which delays metabolism and elimination of many drugs. Drug absorption in neonates is different as a result of slow gastric emptying time. Decreased gastric acid secretion in children younger than 3 years contributes to altered drug absorption. Neonates and infants have a lower concentration of plasma proteins, which can cause toxicity with drugs that are highly bound to proteins. They have less total body fat and more total body water. Therefore, lipid-soluble drugs require smaller doses when less than normal fat is present, and water-soluble drugs can require larger doses because of a greater percentage of body water. As children grow, changes in fat, muscle, body water, and organ maturity can alter the pharmacokinetic effects of drugs. It is the nurse's responsibility to ensure that a safe drug dosage is given and to closely monitor signs and symptoms of adverse reactions to drugs. The purpose of learning how to calculate pediatric drug doses is to ensure that the child receives the correct dose within the therapeutic range.

Oral

Oral pediatric drug delivery often requires the use of a calibrated measuring device, because most drugs for small children are in liquid form. The measuring device can be a small plastic cup, an oral dropper, a measuring spoon, or an oral syringe (Fig. 9–1). Some liquid medications come with their own calibrated drop-

CALIBRATED MEASURING DEVICES

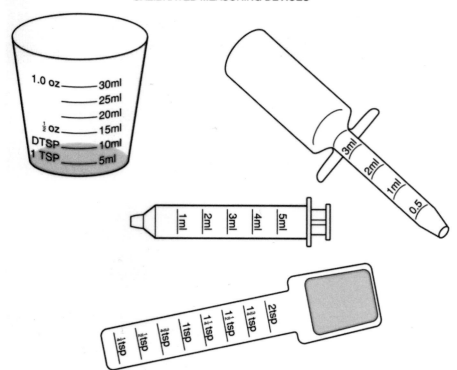

FIGURE 9–1
Calibrated measuring devices.

pers. The type of measuring device chosen depends on the developmental level of the child. For infants and toddlers, the oral syringe and dropper will provide better drug delivery than a small cup. A young child who is cooperative is able to use a small cup or measuring spoon. All liquid medications can be drawn up with a syringe to ensure accuracy and then transferred to a small cup or measuring spoon. It may be necessary to rinse the cup or spoon with water or juice to ensure that the child has received all of the prescribed medication. Avoid giving oral medications to a crying child or infant, because they could easily aspirate the medication. Some chewable medications are available for use in the older child. Because many drugs are enteric coated or in time-release form, the child must be told which medications are to be swallowed and not chewed.

Intramuscular

Intramuscular sites are chosen based on the age and muscle development of the child (Table 9–1). All injections should be given in a manner that minimizes physical and psychosocial trauma. The child must be adequately restrained, if necessary, and provided with a momentary distraction. The procedure must be performed quickly, with comfort measures immediately following.

Intravenous

For children, the maximum amount of IV fluids varies with body weight. Their 24-hour fluid status must be monitored closely to prevent overhydration. The amount of fluid given with IV medication must be considered when planning their 24-hour intake (Table 9–2). After the correct dosage of drug is obtained, it may need further dilution and to be given over a specified time, as mentioned in Chapter 8. Usually, the drug is diluted with 5 to 60 mL of IV fluid, depending on the drug or dosage, placed in a calibrated cylinder, and infused over 20 to 60 minutes, depending on the type of drug. After the drug has infused, the cylinder is flushed with 3 to 20 mL of IV fluid, to ensure that the child has received all of the medication and to prevent admixture. Refer to Chapter 8 for methods of calculating IV infusion rates.

The safety factors that must be considered when administering medications to children are similar to those for adults. See Appendix A for more detailed information on safe nursing practice for drug administration.

TABLE 9–1
Pediatric Guidelines for Intramuscular Injections*

| | MUSCLE GROUP | | | | |
AGE	RECTUS	VASTUS LATERALIS	GLUTEUS MAXIMUS	VENTRO-GLUTEAL	DELTOID
Birth to 2 yr	0.5–1 mL	0.5–1 mL	Not safe	Not safe	Not safe
2 to 3 yr	1 mL	1 mL	1 mL	1 mL	0.5 mL
3 to 7 yr	1.5 mL	1.5 mL	1.5 mL	1.5 mL	0.5 mL
7 to 16 yr	1.5–2 mL	1.5–2 mL	1.5–2 mL	1.5–2 mL	0.5–1 mL
16 yr to adult	2–2.5 mL	2–2.5 mL	2–3 mL	2–3 mL	1–2 mL

* The safe use of all sites is based on normal muscle development and size of the child.

TABLE 9-2
Pediatric Guidelines for 24-Hour Intravenous Fluid Therapy

----

100 mL/kg up to 10 kg body weight
50 mL/kg for the next 5 kg body weight
10 mL/kg after 15 kg body weight

Example: Child's weight 25 kg

$$100 \text{ mL/kg} \times 10 \text{ kg} = 1000 \text{ mL}$$
$$50 \text{ mL/kg} \times 5 \text{ kg} = 250 \text{ mL}$$
$$\underline{10 \text{ mL/kg} \times 10 \text{ kg} = 100 \text{ mL}}$$
$$1350 \text{ mL for 24 hours}$$

PEDIATRIC DRUG CALCULATIONS

The two main methods in determining drug dosages for pediatric drug administration are body weight and body surface area. The first method uses a specific number of milligrams, micrograms, or units for each kilogram of body weight (mg/kg, mcg/kg, U/kg). Usually, drug data for pediatric dosage (mg/kg) are supplied by manufacturers in a drug information insert. Body surface area (BSA), measured by m^2, is considered a more accurate method than body weight. BSA takes into consideration the relation between basal metabolic rate and surface area, which correlates with blood volume, cardiac output, and organ growth and development. Although BSA has primarily been used to calculate the dosage of antineoplastic agents, manufacturers are beginning to include body surface parameters (mg/m^2, mcg/m^2, U/m^2) in drug information.

If the manufacturer does not supply data for pediatric dosing, the child's dosage can be determined from the adult dose. The body surface area formula is used to calculate the pediatric dose. The BSA is considered to be more accurate than previously used formulas such as Clark's, Young's, and Fried's rules. Drug calculations according to the BSA are safer than formulas that rely solely on the child's age or weight. Although the BSA formula has improved the accuracy of drug dosing in infants and children, calculation of drug doses for neonates and preterm infants using this method does not guarantee complete accuracy.

NOTE

If the manufacturer states in the drug information insert that the medication is not for pediatric use the alternative formulas should not be utilized for dosage calculation.

Dosage per Kilogram Body Weight

The following information is needed to calculate the dosage.

a. Physician's order with the name of the drug, the dosage, and the frequency of administration.

b. The child's weight in kilograms:

$$1 \text{ kg} = 2.2 \text{ lb}$$

c. The pediatric dosage as listed by the manufacturer or hospital formulary.

d. Information on how the drug is supplied.

EXAMPLES

PROBLEM 1: **a.** Order: amoxicillin (Amoxil) 60 mg, po, tid.
Child's weight: 12½ lb.

b. Change pounds to kilograms.

$$\frac{12.5}{2.2} = 5.7 \text{ kg}$$

c. Pediatric dosage for children who weigh 20 kg: 20–40 mg/kg/day in three equal doses.

Step 1 Check dosing parameters by multiplying the child's weight by the minimum and maximum daily dose of the drug.

$$20 \text{ mg/kg/day} \times 5.7 \text{ kg} = 114 \text{ mg/day}$$

$$40 \text{ mg/kg/day} \times 5.7 \text{ kg} = 228 \text{ mg/day}$$

Step 2 Multiply the dosage by the frequency to determine the daily dose.
The order for amoxicillin 60 mg, po, tid means that three doses will be given per day.

$$60 \text{ mg} \times 3 = 180 \text{ mg}$$

Because the daily dose of amoxicillin 180 mg falls within the recommended range, it is considered a safe dose.

d. Drug preparation:

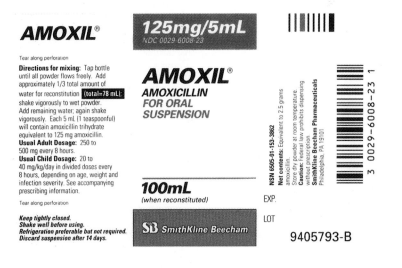

Use either the basic formula, ratio and proportion, or fraction equation.

| | *Basic formula* | **or** | *Ratio and proportion* |

$$\frac{D}{H} \times V = \frac{60 \text{ mg}}{125 \text{ mg}} \times 5 \text{ mL} = 2.4 \text{ mL}$$

$$125 \text{ mg} : 5 \text{ mL} :: 60 \text{ mg} : X \text{ mL}$$
$$125 \text{ X} = 300$$
$$X = 2.4 \text{ mL}$$

Answer: amoxicillin 60 mg, po = 2.4 mL.

PROBLEM 2: **a.** Order: ampicillin 350 mg, IV, q6h. Mix with 20 mL D$_5$/ ¼ NSS, infuse over 20 minutes. Flush with 15 mL. Child weighs 61.5 lb.

    b. Change pounds to kilograms.

$$\frac{61.5}{2.2} = 27.95 \text{ or } 28 \text{ kg}$$

    c. Pediatric dose is 25–50 mg/kg/day in divided doses.

Step 1 Multiply weight by minimum and maximum daily dose.

$$25 \text{ mg} \times 28 \text{ kg} = 700 \text{ mg/day}$$

$$50 \text{ mg} \times 28 \text{ kg} = 1400 \text{ mg/day}$$

Step 2 Multiply the dose by the frequency.

$$350 \text{ mg} \times 4 = 1400 \text{ mg/day}$$

The dose is considered safe because it does not exceed the therapeutic range.

    d. Drug available: When diluted, 500 mg = 2 mL.

```
NDC 0015-7403-20
NSN 6505-00-946-4700
EQUIVALENT TO

500 mg AMPICILLIN
STERILE AMPICILLIN
SODIUM, USP
For IM or IV Use
CAUTION: Federal law prohibits
dispensing without prescription.
```

For IM use, add 1.8 mL diluent (read accompanying circular). Resulting solution contains 250 mg ampicillin per mL. Use solution within 1 hour. This vial contains ampicillin sodium equivalent to 500 mg ampicillin. Usual Dosage: Adults—250 to 500 mg IM q. 6h. READ ACCOMPANYING CIRCULAR for detailed indications, IM or IV dosage and precautions. APOTHECON® A Bristol-Myers Squibb Company Princeton, NJ 08540 USA 7403020DRL-2

Cont: Exp. Date:

Use your selected formula to calculate the dosage.

$$\frac{D}{H} \times V = \frac{350 \text{ mg}}{500 \text{ mg}} \times 2 \text{ mL} = 1.4 \text{ mL}$$ **or** 500 mg : 2 mL :: 350 mg : X mL

$$500 \text{ X} = 700$$
$$X = 1.4 \text{ mL}$$

Answer: Each dose is 1.4 mL.

    e. Amount of fluid to infuse medication.

$$1.4 \text{ mL} + 20 \text{ mL (dilution)} = 21.4 \text{ mL}$$

f. Flow rate calculation (60 gtt/mL set):

$$\frac{\text{amount of solution} \times \text{gtt/mL (set)}}{\text{minutes to administer}} = \text{gtt/min} = \frac{21.4 \text{ mL} \times \overset{3}{\cancel{60}} \text{ gtt/mL}}{\underset{1}{\cancel{20}} \text{ minutes}}$$

$$= 64.2 \text{ gtt/min}$$

g. Total fluid for medication infusion: 21.4 mL + 15 mL (flush) = 36.4 mL

REMEMBER

- *The IV flush (3–20 mL) is part of the total IV fluids necessary for medication administration and must be included in patient intake. The flush is started after IV medication infusion is completed, and it is infused at the same rate.*

- *For a 60 gtt/mL set, the drop per minute rate is the same as the milliliter per minute rate.*

Dosage per Body Surface Area

The following information is needed to calculate the dosage:

a. Physician's order with name of drug, dosage, and time frame or frequency.

b. Child's height, weight in kilograms, and age.

c. Information on how the drug is supplied.

d. Pediatric dosage (in m²) as listed by manufacturer or hospital formulary.

e. Body surface area (BSA) nomogram for children (Fig. 9–1).

EXAMPLE

PROBLEM 1: **a.** Order: methotrexate 50 mg, IV, × 1.
           b. Child's height, weight, age: 134 cm, 32.5 kg, 9 yr.
           c. Pediatric dose: 25–75 mg/m² wk.
           d. Drug preparation: 2.5 mg/mL, 25 mg/mL.
           e. Body surface area nomogram for children: The child's height (134 cm) and weight (32.5 kg) intersect at 1.11 m² BSA.

Multiply the BSA, 1.11 m², by the minimum and maximum dose. (Substitute BSA for weight.)

$$25 \text{ mg/m}^2 \times 1.11 \text{ m}^2 = 28.0 \text{ mg}$$

$$75 \text{ mg/m}^2 \times 1.11 \text{ m}^2 = 83.0 \text{ mg}$$

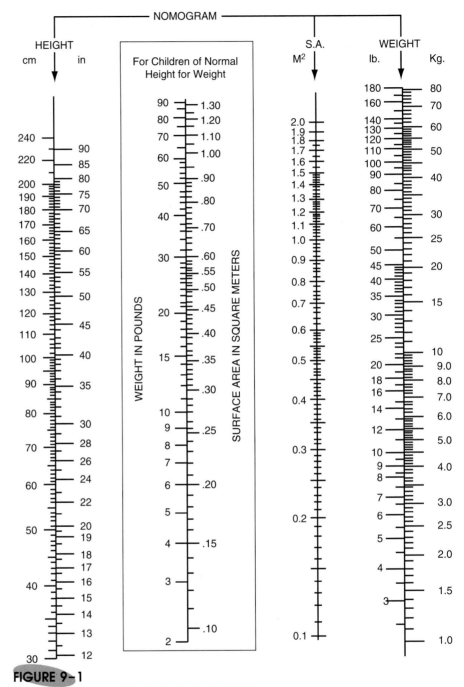

FIGURE 9–1

West nomogram: for infants and children.

Directions: (1) Find height. (2) Find weight. (3) Draw a straight line connecting the height and the weight, and where the line intersects on the SA column is the body surface area (m²). (Modified from data of E. Boyd and C. D. West, in Behrman, R. E., and Vaughan, V. C.: Nelson Textbook of Pediatrics, 14th ed. Philadelphia, W. B. Saunders Co., 1992.)

This dose is considered safe because it is within the therapeutic range for the child's body surface area.

> **f.** Calculate drug dose: to determine the amount of drug to be administered, either formula can be used.

$$\frac{D}{H} \times V = \frac{50 \text{ mg}}{25 \text{ mg}} \times 1 \text{ mL} = 2 \text{ mL} \quad \textbf{or} \quad 25 \text{ mg} : 1 \text{ mL} : : = 50 \text{ mg} : X \text{ mL}$$

$$25 X = 50$$
$$X = 2 \text{ mL}$$

Answer: methotrexate 50 mg = 2 mL.

Practice Problems

With the following dosage problems for oral, IM, and IV administration, determine if the ordered dose is safe and how much of the drug should be given.

I. Oral

1. Child with rheumatic fever.
Order: penicillin V potassium 250 mg, po, q8h.
Child's weight: 45 lb.
Pediatric dose: 25–50 mg/kg/day.
Drug available:

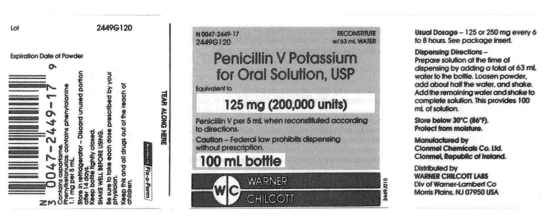

2. Child with seizures.
Order: Phenobarbital 25 mg, po, bid.
Child's weight: 7.2 kg.
Pediatric dose: 5–7 mg/kg/day.
Drug available: phenobarbital 20 mg/5 mL.

3. Child with lower respiratory tract infection.
Order: cloxacillin 100 mg, po, qid.
Child's weight: 17 lb.
Pediatric dose: 50 mg/kg/day.
Drug available:

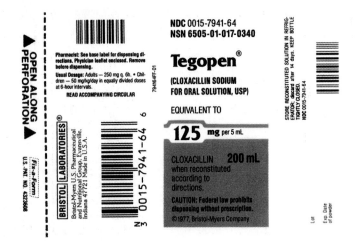

4. Child with pain.
Order: codeine 7.5 mg, po, q4h, PRN × 6 doses/day.
Child's height and weight: 43 inches, 50 lb.
Pediatric dose: 100 mg/m²/day (see Fig. 9–1).
Drug available: codeine 15-mg tablets.

5. Child with seizures.
Order: Zarontin 125 mg, po, bid.
Child's weight: 13 kg.
Pediatric dose: 20 mg/kg/day.
Drug available:

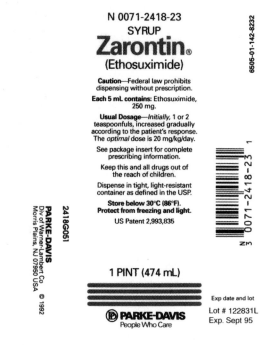

6. Child with seizures.
Order: Dilantin 40 mg, po, bid.

Child's weight: 6.7 kg.
Pediatric dose: 5–7 mg/kg/day.
Drug available:

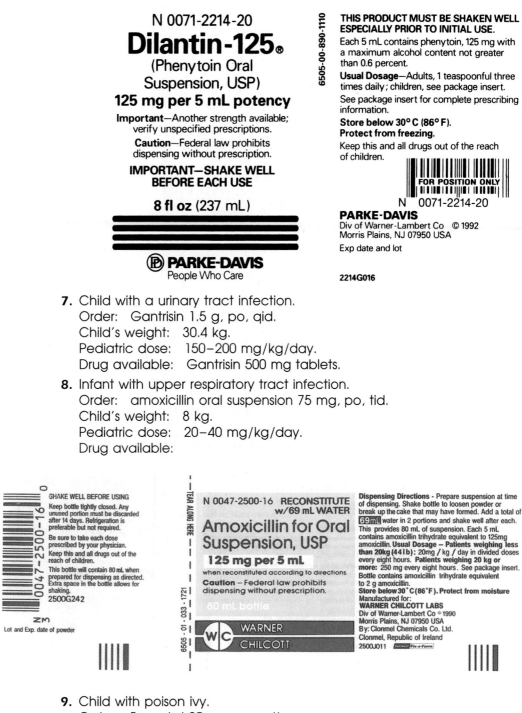

N 0071-2214-20

Dilantin-125®

(Phenytoin Oral
Suspension, USP)

125 mg per 5 mL potency

Important—Another strength available;
verify unspecified prescriptions.

Caution—Federal law prohibits
dispensing without prescription.

**IMPORTANT—SHAKE WELL
BEFORE EACH USE**

8 fl oz (237 mL)

Ⓟ **PARKE-DAVIS**
People Who Care

6505-00-890-1110

**THIS PRODUCT MUST BE SHAKEN WELL
ESPECIALLY PRIOR TO INITIAL USE.**

Each 5 mL contains phenytoin, 125 mg with
a maximum alcohol content not greater
than 0.6 percent.

Usual Dosage—Adults, 1 teaspoonful three
times daily; children, see package insert.

See package insert for complete prescribing
information.

**Store below 30° C (86° F).
Protect from freezing.**

Keep this and all drugs out of the reach
of children.

FOR POSITION ONLY

N   0071-2214-20

PARKE-DAVIS
Div of Warner-Lambert Co © 1992
Morris Plains, NJ 07950 USA

Exp date and lot

2214G016

7. Child with a urinary tract infection.
Order: Gantrisin 1.5 g, po, qid.
Child's weight: 30.4 kg.
Pediatric dose: 150–200 mg/kg/day.
Drug available: Gantrisin 500 mg tablets.

8. Infant with upper respiratory tract infection.
Order: amoxicillin oral suspension 75 mg, po, tid.
Child's weight: 8 kg.
Pediatric dose: 20–40 mg/kg/day.
Drug available:

SHAKE WELL BEFORE USING

Keep bottle tightly closed. Any
unused portion must be discarded
after 14 days. Refrigeration is
preferable but not required.

Be sure to take each dose
prescribed by your physician.
Keep this and all drugs out of the
reach of children.

This bottle will contain 80 mL when
prepared for dispensing as directed.
Extra space in the bottle allows for
shaking.
2500G242

Lot and Exp. date of powder

TEAR ALONG HERE

6505 - 01 - 033 - 1721

N 0047-2500-16 **RECONSTITUTE
w/69 mL WATER**

Amoxicillin for Oral Suspension, USP

125 mg per 5 mL

when reconstituted according to directions.

Caution – Federal law prohibits
dispensing without prescription.

80 mL bottle

W/C WARNER
CHILCOTT

Dispensing Directions - Prepare suspension at time
of dispensing. Shake bottle to loosen powder or
break up the cake that may have formed. Add a total of
69 mL water in 2 portions and shake well after each.
This provides 80 mL of suspension. Each 5 mL
contains amoxicillin trihydrate equivalent to 125mg
amoxicillin. **Usual Dosage – Patients weighing less
than 20kg (44 lb):** 20mg / kg / day in divided doses
every eight hours. **Patients weighing 20 kg or
more:** 250 mg every eight hours. See package insert.
Bottle contains amoxicillin trihydrate equivalent
to 2 g amoxicillin.
Store below 30˚C (86˚F). Protect from moisture
Manufactured for:
WARNER CHILCOTT LABS
Div of Warner-Lambert Co © 1990
Morris Plains, NJ 07950 USA
By: Clonmel Chemicals Co. Ltd.
Clonmel, Republic of Ireland
2500J011

9. Child with poison ivy.
Order: Benadryl 25 mg, po, q6h.
Child's weight: 25 kg.

Pediatric dose: 5 mg/kg/day.
Drug available: Benadryl 12.5 mg/5 mL.

10. Child with cystic fibrosis exposed to influenza A.
Order: Symmetrel 25 mg, po, tid.
Child's weight: 14 kg.
Pediatric dose: 4–8 mg/kg/day.
Drug available:

NDC 0056-0205-16   NDC 0056-0205-16

DUPONT PHARMACEUTICALS
SYMMETREL®
(amantadine hydrochloride)

DUPONT PHARMACEUTICALS
SYMMETREL®
(amantadine hydrochloride)

Each teaspoonful
(5 ml) contains:
Amantadine
hydrochloride .... 50 mg

CAUTION: Federal law prohibits
dispensing without prescription.
DOSAGE: For dosage and full
prescribing information read
accompanying product insert.

ONE PINT (480 ml) SYRUP

DuPont Pharmaceuticals
E.I. du Pont de Nemours & Co.
Wilmington, Delaware 19898

Made and Printed in U.S.A.   7064/BJ

Each teaspoonful
(5 ml) contains:
Amantadine
hydrochloride .... 50 mg

CAUTION: Federal law prohibits
dispensing without prescription.
DOSAGE: For dosage and full
prescribing information read
accompanying product insert.
Dispense in a tight container as
defined in the U.S.P.
KEEP TIGHTLY CLOSED
Store at controlled room temperature (59°-86° F, 15°-30° C).

ONE PINT (480 ml) SYRUP

3 0056-0205-16 8

Lot: ECIMEN
Exp:

II. Intramuscular

11. Child with nausea postsurgery.
Order: Phenergan 20 mg, IM, q6h.
Child's weight: 45 kg.
Pediatric dose: 0.25–0.5 mg/kg/dose, repeat 4–6 hr.
Drug available: Phenergan 25 mg/mL.

12. Child has strep throat.
Order: Bicillin C-R, 1,000,000 U, IM, × 1.
Child's weight: 44 lb.
Pediatric dose: 30–60 lb: 900,000–1,200,000 U daily.
Drug available: Bicillin C-R 1,200,000 U/2 mL.

13. Child receiving preoperative medication.
Order: hydroxyzine (Vistaril) 25 mg, IM.
Child's height and weight: 47 inches, 45 lb.
Pediatric dose: 30 mg/m^2.
Drug available: Vistaril 25 mg/mL.

14. Child receiving preoperative medication.
Order: atropine 0.2 mg, IM.
Child's weight: 12 kg.
Pediatric dose: 24–40 lb/0.2 mg.

Drug available:

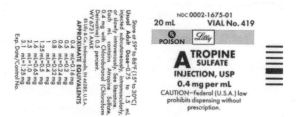

15. Child with cancer.
Order: methotrexate 50 mg, IM, q weekly.
Child's height and weight: 56 inches, 100 lb.
Pediatric dose: 25–75 mg/m^2/wk.
Drug available: methotrexate 2.5 mg/mL; 25 mg/mL; 100 mg/mL.

III. Intravenous

16. Adolescent with progressive hip pain secondary to rheumatoid arthritis.
Order: morphine sulfate 2.5 mg, IV piggyback, in 10 mL NSS over 5 minutes. Flush with 5 mL.
Child's weight: 50 kg.
Pediatric dose: 50–100 mcg/kg/dose for IV.
Drug available:

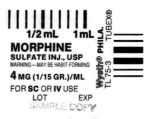

17. Treatment to reverse postoperative narcotic depression.
Order: Narcan 0.3 mg, IV push.
Child's weight: 32 kg.
Pediatric dose: 0.005–0.01 mg/kg.
Drug available:

18. Infant with sepsis.
   Order: Amikin 40 mg, IV, q12h, in D₅W 5 mL, over 20 minutes.
   Flush with 3 mL.
   Child's weight: 5.3 kg.
   Pediatric dose: 15 mg/kg/day.
   Drug available:

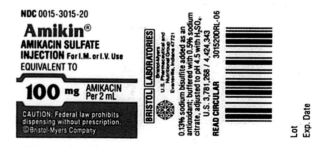

19. Child with head trauma.
   Order: Decadron 2 mg, IV, q6h, in D₅W 10 mL, over 15 minutes.
   Flush with 5 mL.
   Child's weight and age: 10.1 kg, 16 months.
   Pediatric dose: 0.4 mg/kg/day in divided doses.
   Drug available:

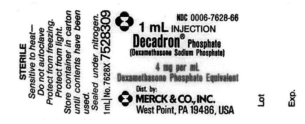

20. Child with pneumonia.
   Order: ampicillin 500 mg, IV, q6h, in D₅W 20 mL, over 30 minutes.
   Flush with 3 mL.
   Child's weight: 5.6 kg.
   Pediatric dose: 300 mg/kg/day.
   Drug available:

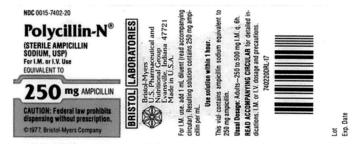

21. Child with sepsis.
   Order: gentamicin 10 mg, IV, q8h, in D₅W, 4 mL over 30 minutes.
   Flush with 3 mL.
   Child's height, weight, age: 21 inches, 4 kg, 1 month.

Pediatric dose: >7 days old: 5–7.5 mg/kg/day, 3–4 divided doses.
Drug available: gentamicin 10 mg/mL.

22. Child with postoperative wound infection.
Order: cefazolin 185 mg, IV, q6h, in D_5W 20 mL, over 20 minutes. Flush with 15 mL.
Child's weight: 15 kg.
Pediatric dose: 25–50 mg/kg/day.
Drug available:

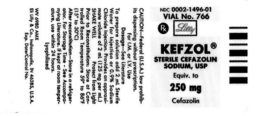

23. Child with wound infection after spinal fusion.
Order: nafcillin 250 mg, IV, q6h, in D_5W 20 cc, over 30 minutes. Flush with 15 mL.
Child's weight: 40 kg.
Pediatric dose: 25 mg/kg/day.
Drug available:

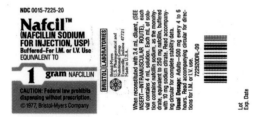

24. Child with congestive heart failure.
Order: digoxin 40 mcg, IV, bid, in NSS 2 mL, over 1 minute.
Child's weight and age: 6 lb, 1 month.
Pediatric dose: 2 weeks to 2 years: 25–50 mcg/kg.
Drug available: digoxin 0.1 mg/mL.

25. Child with lymphoma.
Order: Cytoxan 180 mg, IV, in $D_5\frac{1}{2}$ NSS, 300 mL over 3 hours, no flush to follow.
Child's weight and height: 16 kg, 75 cm.
Pediatric dose: 300 mg/m^2/day.
Drug available:

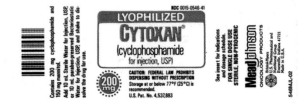

26. Child with severe respiratory infection.
Order: kanamycin (Kantrex) 60 mg, IV, q8h.
Drug available:

NDC 0015-3512-20
6505-00-926-9202
Kantrex®
KANAMYCIN SULFATE
PEDIATRIC INJECTION
FOR I.M. OR I.V. USE
EQUIVALENT TO
75 mg KANAMYCIN
per 2 ml

BRISTOL LABORATORIES
Div of Bristol-Myers Company
Syracuse, NY 13221-4755

0.099% sodium bisulfite added as an antioxidant, buffered with 0.33% sodium citrate. • Adjusted to pH 4.5 with H₂SO₄. • Kantrex Pediatric Injection should not be physically mixed with other antibacterial agents. **READ ACCOMPANYING CIRCULAR**
CAUTION: Federal law prohibits dispensing without prescription.
©Bristol Laboratories
351220DRL-13

MAXIMUM DOSE: 15 MG/KG/DAY

Lot

Exp. Date

Child's weight and age: 26 lb, 12 months.
Pediatric dose parameters: 15 mg/kg/day q8–12h, not to exceed 1.5 g per day.

a. How many mL of kanamycin will the child receive per q8h?

_____

b. How many mL of kanamycin will the child receive per day?

_____

c. Is the drug dose within safe parameters? _____

27. Child with severe systemic infection.
Order: tobramycin (Nebcin) 15 mg, IV, q6h.
Drug available:

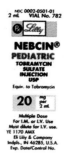

NDC 0002-0501-01
2 mL   VIAL No. 782

℞ *Lilly*

NEBCIN®
PEDIATRIC
TOBRAMYCIN
SULFATE
INJECTION
USP
Equiv. to Tobramycin

20 mg per 2 mL

Multiple Dose
For I.M. or I.V. Use
Must dilute for I.V. use.
YE 1170 AMX
Eli Lilly & Company
Indpls., IN 46285, U.S.A.
Exp. Date/Control No.

Child's weight and age: 10 kg, 18 months.
Pediatric dose parameters: 6–7.5 mg/kg/day in 3 or 4 divided doses.

a. How many mL of tobramycin would you give?

_____

b. Is the drug dose within safe parameters?

_____

PEDIATRIC DOSAGE FROM ADULT DOSAGE

Body Surface Area Formula

The following information is needed to calculate the pediatric dosage using the BSA formula:

a. Physician's order with the name of the drug, the dosage, and the time frame or frequency.

b. The child's height and weight.

c. A body surface area nomogram for children.

d. The adult drug dosage.

e. The body surface area formula:

$$\frac{\text{surface area (m}^2)}{1.73 \text{ m}^2} \times \text{adult dose} = \text{child's dose}$$

EXAMPLE

PROBLEM 1: **a.** erythromycin 80 mg, po, qid.
           b. Child's height is 34 inches and weight is 28.5 lb.

Note: *Height and weight do not have to be converted to the metric system.*

       c. Height (34 inches) and weight (28.5 lb) intersect the nomogram at 0.57 m². See BSA nomogram, Figure 9–1.
       d. The adult drug dosage is 1000 mg/24 hr.
       e. Body surface area formula:

$$\frac{\text{surface area (m}^2)}{173 \text{ m}^2} \times \text{adult dose} = \frac{0.57 \text{ m}^2}{1.73 \text{ m}^2} \times 100$$
$$= 0.33 \times 1000$$
$$= 330 \text{ mg/24 hr}$$

Dose frequency:

$$330 \text{ mg} \div 4 \text{ doses} = 82.5$$

or

80 mg per dose

Dosage is safe.

$$80 \text{ mg} \times 4 \text{ times per day} = 320 \text{ mg/day}$$

Age Rules

Fried's rule and Young's rule are two methods for determining pediatric drug doses based on the child's age. Fried's rule is primarily used for children younger than 1 year of age, whereas Young's rule is used for children between 2 and 12 years of age. In current practice, these rules are infrequently used. Because the maturational development of infants and children is variable, age cannot be an accurate basis for drug dosing.

Fried's Rule:

$$\frac{\text{Age in months}}{150} \times \text{adult dose} = \text{infant's dose}$$

Young's Rule:

$$\frac{\text{child's age in years}}{\text{age in years} + 12} \times \text{adult dose} = \text{child's dose}$$

Body Weight Rule

Clark's rule is another method to derive a pediatric dosage based on the child's weight in pounds and the average adult weight of 150 lb. Population studies have shown an increase in the average weight of adults; therefore, 150 lb is an accurate constant. Using the fixed constant in Clark's rule can lead to the underdosing of infants. Clark's rule is being phased out as a method for determining drug dosage in children.

Clark's Rule:

$$\frac{\text{child's weight in pounds}}{150 \text{ lb}} \times \text{adult dose} = \text{child's dose}$$

NOTE

The age and weight rules should not be used if a pediatric dose is provided by the manufacturer.

ANSWERS

I. Oral

1. Pounds to kilograms: $\dfrac{45 \text{ lb}}{2.2 \text{ lb/kg}} = 20.4 \text{ kg}$

Dosage parameters: 25 mg/kg/day × 20.4 kg = 510 mg/day
50 mg/kg/day × 20.4 kg = 1020 mg/day
Dosage frequency: 250 mg × 3 = 750 mg
Dosage is safe.

$$\frac{D}{H} \times V = \frac{250 \text{ mg}}{125 \text{ mg}} \times 5 \text{ mL} = 10 \text{ mL}$$

2. Dosage parameters: 5 mg/kg/day × 7.2 kg = 36 mg/day
7 mg/kg/day × 7.2 kg = 50.4 mg/day
Dose frequency: 25 mg × 2 = 50 mg
Dosage is safe.

$$\frac{D}{H} \times V = \frac{25 \text{ mg}}{20 \text{ mg}} \times 5 \text{ mL} = 6.25 \text{ mL/dose}$$

3. Dosage parameters: 50 mg/kg/day × 8 kg = 400 mg/day
Dosage frequency: 100 mg × 4 = 400 mg
Dosage is safe.

$$\frac{D}{H} \times V = \frac{100 \text{ mg}}{125 \text{ mg}} \times 5 \text{ mL} = 4 \text{ mL}$$

4. Height and weight intersect at 0.84 m^2.
Dosage parameters: 100 mg/0.84 m^2/day = 84 mg/day
Dose frequency: 84 mg/day ÷ 6 = 14 mg/dose
Dosage is safe.

$$\frac{D}{H} \times V = \frac{7.5 \text{ mg}}{15 \text{ mg}} \times 1 = 0.50 \text{ or } \frac{1}{2} \text{ tablet}$$

5. Dosage parameters: 20 mg/kg/day × 13 kg = 260 mg/day
Dosage frequency: 125 mg × 2 = 250 mg/day
Dosage is safe.

$$\frac{D}{H} \times V = \frac{125 \text{ mg}}{250 \text{ mg}} \times 5 \text{ mL} = 2.5 \text{ mL}$$

6. Dosage parameters: 5 mg/kg/day × 6.7 kg = 33.5 mg/day
                                       7 mg/kg/day × 6.7 kg = 46.9 mg/day
Dose frequency: 40 mg × 2 = 80 mg
Dosage exceeds the therapeutic range. Dosage is *not* safe.

7. Dosage parameters: 150 mg/kg/day × 30.4 = 4560 mg or 4.5 g
                                       200 mg/kg/day × 30.4 = 6080 mg or 6.1 g
Dose frequency: 1.5 g × 4 = 6.0 g or 6000 mg
Dosage is safe.

$$\frac{D}{H} = \frac{1500 \text{ mg}}{500 \text{ mg}} = 3 \text{ tablets per dose}$$

8. Dosage parameters: 20 mg/kg/day × 8 kg = 160 mg/day
                                       40 mg/kg/day × 8 kg = 320 mg/day
Dosage frequency: 75 mg × 3 = 225 mg
Dosage is safe.

$$\frac{D}{H} \times V = \frac{75 \text{ mg}}{125 \text{ mg}} \times 5 \text{ mL} = 3 \text{ mL}$$

9. Dosage parameters: 5 mg/kg/day × 25 kg = 125 mg/day
Dosage frequency: 25 mg × 4 = 100 mg/day
Dosage is safe.

$$\frac{D}{H} \times V = \frac{25 \text{ mg}}{12.5 \text{ mg}} \times 5 \text{ mL} = 10 \text{ mL}$$

10. Dosage parameters: 4 mg/kg/day × 14 kg = 56 mg/day
                                        8 mg/kg/day × 14 kg = 112 mg/day
Dose frequency: 25 mg × 3 = 75 mg
Dosage is safe.

$$\frac{D}{H} \times V = \frac{25 \text{ mg}}{50 \text{ mg}} \times 5 \text{ mL} = 2.5 \text{ mL/dose}$$

II. Intramuscular

11. Dosage parameters: 0.25/kg/dose × 45 kg = 11.25 mg/dose
                                        0.5/kg/dose × 45 kg = 22.5 mg/dose
Dose frequency: 20 mg IM/dose
Dosage is safe.

$$\frac{D}{H} \times V = \frac{20 \text{ mg}}{25 \text{ mg}} \times 1 = 0.8 \text{ mL}$$

12. Dosage parameters:
Child's weight is 44 lb, which falls in the 30–60 lb pediatric dose range.
Dose frequency:
The one time dose of 1,000,000 U falls within the pediatric dose range.
Dosage is safe.

$$\frac{D}{H} \times V = \frac{1,000,000 \text{ U}}{1,200,000 \text{ U}} \times 2 = 1.6 \text{ mL}$$

13. Height and weight intersect at 0.82 m².
Dosage parameters: 30 mg/m² × 0.82 m² = 24.6 mg or 25 mg
Dose frequency: 25 mg, IM
Dosage is safe.

$$\frac{D}{H} \times V = \frac{25 \text{ mg}}{25 \text{ mg}} \times 1 = 1.0 \text{ mL}$$

14. Kilograms to pounds: 12 kg × 2.2 lb/kg = 26.4 lb
Dosage is safe.

$$\frac{D}{H} \times V = \frac{0.2}{0.4} \times 1 = 0.5 \text{ mL}$$

15. Height and weight intersect at 1.38 m².
Dosage parameters: 25 mg/m²/wk × 1.38 m² = 34.5 mg/wk
                     75 mg/m²/wk × 1.38 m² = 103.5 mg/wk
Dose frequency: 50 mg/wk IM
Dosage is safe.

$$\frac{D}{H} \times V = \frac{50}{100} \text{ mg} \times 1 = 0.5 \text{ mL}$$

III. Intravenous

16. Dosage parameters: 50 mcg/kg/dose × 50 kg = 2500 mcg/dose or
2.5 mg/dose
100 mcg/kg/dose × 50 kg = 5000 mcg/dose
or 5 mg/dose
Dosage is safe.

$$\frac{D}{H} \times V = \frac{2.5}{4} \times 1 = 0.62 \text{ or } 0.6 \text{ mL}$$

Amount of fluid to infuse: 0.6 mL + 10 mL = 10.6 mL

$$\frac{10.6 \text{ mL} \times \overset{12}{\cancel{60}} \text{ gtt/mL}}{\underset{1}{\cancel{5} \text{ minutes}}} = 127.2 \text{ gtt/min}$$

Total fluid for medication infusion: 10.6 mL + 5 mL = 15.6 mL.

17. Dosage parameters: 0.005 mg/kg/dose × 32 kg = 0.16 mg
                            0.01 mg/kg/dose × 32 kg = 0.32 mg
Dosage is safe.

$$\frac{D}{H} \times V = \frac{0.3}{0.4} \times 1 = 0.75 \text{ mL}$$

18. Dosage parameters: 15 mg/kg/day × 5.3 = 79.5 mg/day
Dosage frequency: 40 mg IV × 2 = 80 mg
79.5 mg is rounded off to 80 mg. The dosage is safe.

$$\frac{D}{H} \times V = \frac{40 \text{ mg}}{100 \text{ mg}} \times 2 = 0.8 \text{ mL}$$

Amount of fluid to infuse: 0.8 mL + 5 mL = 5.8 mL

$$\frac{5.8 \text{ mL} \times \overset{3}{\cancel{60}} \text{ gtt/mL}}{\underset{1}{\cancel{20}} \text{ minutes}} = 17.4 \text{ gtt/min}$$

Total fluid for medication infusion: 5.8 mL + 3 mL = 8.8 mL.

19. Dosage parameters: 0.4 mg/kg/day × 10.1 kg = 4 mg/day
Dose frequency:

$$2 \text{ mg} \times 4 \text{ times/day} = 8 \text{ mg per day}$$

or

$$4 \text{ mg} \div 4 \text{ doses} = 1 \text{ mg per dose}$$

Dose exceeds therapeutic range of 1 mg per dose. Dosage is *not* safe.

20. Dosage parameters: 300 mg × 5.6 kg = 1680 mg/day
Dose frequency: 1680 mg ÷ 4 doses = 420 mg per dose
Dose exceeds therapeutic range of 420 mg per dose. Dosage is *not* safe.

21. Dosage parameters: 5 mg/kg/day × 4 kg = 20 mg/day
                             7.5 mg/kg/day × 4 kg = 30 mg/day
Dose frequency: 10 mg × 3 times/day = 30 mg
Dosage is safe.

$$\frac{D}{H} \times V = \frac{10 \text{ mg}}{10 \text{ mg}} \times 1 \text{ mL} = 1 \text{ mL}$$

Amount of fluid to infuse: 1 mL + 4 mL = 5 mL

$$\frac{5 \text{ mL} \times \overset{2}{\cancel{60}} \text{ gtt/mL}}{\underset{1}{\cancel{30}} \text{ minutes}} = 10 \text{ gtt/min}$$

Total fluid for medication infusion: 5 mL + 3 mL = 8 mL

22. Dosage parameters: 25 mg/kg/day × 15 kg = 375 mg/day
                             50 mg/kg/day × 15 kg = 750 mg/day
Dosage frequency: 185 mg × 4 = 740 mg/day
Dosage is safe.

$$\frac{D}{H} \times V = \frac{185 \text{ mg}}{125 \text{ mg}} \times 1 \text{ mL} = 1.48 \text{ or } 1.5 \text{ mL}$$

Amount of fluid to infuse: 1.5 mL + 20 mL = 21.5 mL

$$\frac{21.5 \text{ mL} \times \overset{3}{\cancel{60}} \text{ gtt/mL}}{\underset{1}{\cancel{20}} \text{ minutes}} = 64.5 \text{ gtt/min}$$

Total fluid for medication infusion: 21.5 mL + 15 mL = 36.5 mL

23. Dosage parameters: 25 mg/kg/day × 40 kg = 1000 mg
Dosage frequency: 250 mg × 4 = 1000 mg/day
Dosage is safe.

$$\frac{D}{H} \times V = \frac{250}{1000} \times 4 = 1 \text{ mL}$$

Amount of fluid to infuse: 1 mL + 20 mL = 21 mL

$$\frac{21 \text{ mL} \times \overset{2}{\cancel{60}} \text{ gtt/mL (set)}}{\underset{1}{\cancel{30}} \text{ minutes}} = 42 \text{ gtt/min}$$

Total fluid for medication infusion: 21 mL + 15 mL = 36 mL

24. Dosage parameters: 25 mcg/kg/day × 2.72 kg = 68 mcg
        50 mcg/kg/day × 2.72 kg = 136 mcg
Dosage frequency: 40 mcg × 2 = 80 mcg
Dosage is safe.

$$\frac{D}{H} \times V = \frac{40 \text{ mcg}}{100 \text{ mcg}} \times 1 = 0.4 \text{ mL}$$

25. Height and weight intersect at 0.6 m^2.
Dosage parameters: 300 mg/m^2/day × 0.6 m^2 = 180 mg/day
Dosage is safe.

$$\frac{D}{H} \times V = \frac{180 \text{ mg}}{200 \text{ mg}} \times 10 \text{ mL} = 9 \text{ mL}$$

Total amount of fluid to infuse: 9 mL + 300 mL = 309 mL

$$\frac{309 \text{ mL}}{3 \text{ hr}} = 103 \text{ mL/hr or } 103 \text{ gtt/min with a 60 gtt/mL set}$$

26. a. $\dfrac{60}{75} \times 2 \text{ mL} = \dfrac{120}{75} = 1.6 \text{ mL}$ **or**   75 mg : 2 mL : : 60 mg : X
                75 X = 120
                X = 1.6 mL of
                        kanamycin

b. 4.8 mL/day

c. Dosage parameters: 15 mg × 12 kg = 180 mg/day
        60 mg × 3 (q8h) = 180 mg/day
Drug dose per day is within safe parameters.

27. a. $\dfrac{15}{\underset{10}{\cancel{20}}} \times \overset{1}{\cancel{2}} \text{ mL} = \dfrac{15}{10}$ **or**   20 mg : 2 mL : : 15 mg : X
        = 1.5 mL of Nebcin   20 X = 30
                X = 1.5 mL of Nebcin

b. Pediatric dose parameters: 6 mg/10 kg/day = 60 mg/day
        7.5 mg/10 kg/day = 75 mg/day
        15 mg × 4 (q6h) = 60 mg/day
Drug dose per day is within safe parameters.

Critical Care

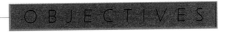

O B J E C T I V E S

- Calculate the prescribed concentration of a drug in solution.
- Identify the units of measure designated for the amount of drug in solution.
- Describe the four determinants of infusion rates.
- Calculate the concentration of drug per unit time for a specific body weight.
- Recognize the variables needed for the basic fractional formula.
- Describe how the titration factor is used when infusion rates are changed.
- Recognize the methods of determining the total amount of drug infused over time.
- Identify the advantages and disadvantages of the "factor of 15" method.

Medication administration has become more individualized in the specialty areas. Often it is necessary to calculate the patient's dose in micrograms per kilogram of body weight per minute or in units per hour. As the patient's condition changes, medications may be added or discontinued, which may necessitate calculating the total amount of drug administered over a short period of time. Administration of potent drugs in milligrams, micrograms, or units per body weight or unit time requires extreme accuracy in calculations. Research studies have shown a high incidence of error in drug calculations among nurses and physicians. Many institutions have initiated policies of drug infusion standardization, especially for concentration of solution. Drug manufacturers provide dosage administration charts for quick reference to initiate drug treatment. However, most charts use ranges of weight or rates, which prevents individualization of drug doses. Basic knowledge of calculations, used to determine administration of individualized dosage, can validate the accuracy of the physician's order and verify the dosage chosen from an administration chart.

Physicians determine the amount of drug to be mixed in the infusate (solution) and designate infusion rates or the dosage per kilogram of body weight per unit time. Some institutions have their own guidelines for preparation of medication in the critical care areas, but the administration and calculation of the actual dose is a nursing function.

The mathematical skills needed to solve problems in this chapter include the knowledge of proper and improper fractions, cancellation of units, ratio and proportion, and conversion to the metric system.

CALCULATING AMOUNT OF DRUG OR CONCENTRATION OF A SOLUTION

The first step in administering a medication is to determine the concentration of the solution, which is the amount of drug in each milliliter of solution. This is written as units per milliliter, milligrams per milliliter, or micrograms per milliliter and must be calculated for each problem. For all problems, remember to convert to like units before solving.

Calculating Units per Milliliter

EXAMPLE

PROBLEM: Infuse heparin 5000 U in D_5W 250 mL at 30 mL/hr. What will be the concentration of heparin in each milliliter of D_5W?

Method: units/mL

Set up a ratio and proportion. Solve for X.

$$5000 \text{ U} : 250 \text{ mL} : : \text{X U} : \text{mL}$$

$$250 \text{ X} = 5000$$
$$\text{X} = 20 \text{ U}$$

Answer: The D_5W with heparin will have a concentration of 20 U/mL of solution.

Calculating Milligrams per Milliliter

EXAMPLE

PROBLEM: Infuse lidocaine 2 g in 500 mL D_5W at 2 mg/min. What will be the concentration of lidocaine in each milliliter of D_5W?

Method: mg/mL

Convert grams to milligrams. Set up a ratio and proportion and solve for X.

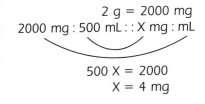

$$2\ g = 2000\ mg$$
$$2000\ mg : 500\ mL :: X\ mg : mL$$

$$500\ X = 2000$$
$$X = 4\ mg$$

Answer: The D_5W with lidocaine has a concentration of 4 mg/mL of solution.

Calculating Micrograms per Milliliter

EXAMPLE

PROBLEM: Infuse dobutamine 250 mg in 500 mL D_5W at 650 mcg/min. What is the concentration of dobutamine in each milliliter of D_5W?

Method: mcg/mL

Convert milligrams to micrograms. Set up a ratio and proportion and solve for X.

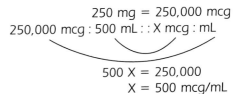

$$250\ mg = 250,000\ mcg$$
$$250,000\ mcg : 500\ mL :: X\ mcg : mL$$

$$500\ X = 250,000$$
$$X = 500\ mcg/mL$$

Answer: The D_5W with dobutamine will have a concentration of 500 mcg/mL of solution.

1. Practice Problems: Calculating Concentration of a Solution

1. Infuse heparin 10,000 U in 250 mL D_5W at 30 mL/hr.

_____

2. Infuse aminophylline 250 mg in 500 mL D_5W at 50 mL/hr.

_____

3. Order: regular insulin 100 U in 500 mL NSS at 30 mL/hr.

_____

4. Order: lidocaine 1 g in 100 mL D_5W at 30 mL/hr.

_____

5. Order: norepinephrine 4 mg in 500 mL D_5W at 15 mL/hr.

_____

6. Order: dopamine 500 mg in 250 mL D_5W at 10 mL/hr.

_____

7. Order: dobutamine 400 mg in 250 mL D_5W at 20 mL/hr.

_____

8. Order: Isuprel 2 mg in 250 mL D_5W at 10 mL/hr.

_____

9. Order: streptokinase 750,000 U in 50 mL D_5W over 30 minutes.

_____

10. Order: nitroprusside 50 mg in 500 mL D_5W at 50 mcg/min.

_____

11. Order: aminophylline 1 g in 250 mL D_5W at 20 mL/hr.

_____

12. Order: Pronestyl 2 g in 250 mL D_5W at 16 mL/hr.

_____

13. Order: heparin 25,000 U in 250 mL D_5W at 5 mL/hr.

_____

14. Order: Aminophyllin 1 g in 500 mL at 40 cc/hr.

_____

15. Order: nitroglycerin 50 mg in 250 mL D_5W at 50 mcg/min.

_____

CALCULATING INFUSION RATE FOR CONCENTRATION AND VOLUME PER UNIT TIME

The second step for administering medication is to calculate the *infusion rate* of drug per *unit time*. Infusion rates can mean two things: the rate of volume (mL) given or the rate of concentration (units, mg, mcg) administered. Unit time means per hour or per minute. For drugs administered by continuous infusion, the four most important determinants are the concentration per hour and minute and the volume per hour and minute. Infusion rates of potent drugs are usually part of the physician's order and may be stated in concentration or volume per unit time.

The widespread use of microdrip IV administration sets for the delivery of potent drugs and the use of volumetric infusion pumps, which are calibrated in milliliters per hour, limit the need for calculating infusion rates in drops per minute. As noted in Chapter 8, when using the microdrip administration set, the milliliter per hour rate corresponds to the drop per minute rate. The concentration per volume per unit time is the most accurate and safest method of drug administration. Potent drugs should always be administered with volumetric infusion pumps in a closely monitored environment.

Complete infusion rates for volume and concentration are given in the examples and practice problems. In clinical practice, not all the data are needed for each drug. For heparin, the concentration per minute is not as vital as the concentration per hour, whereas for vasoactive drugs such as dobutamine, the concentration per minute is essential information and the concentration per hour is not. The same methods of calculation are used for both drugs and the same information can be obtained. Knowledge of pharmacology and clinical practice will help in determining what is the most useful data.

Concentration and Volume per Hour and Minute with a Drug in Units

EXAMPLE

PROBLEM: Infuse heparin 5000 U in D_5W 250 mL at 30 mL/hr.

Concentration of solution is 20 units/mL
(Also note that volume/hr is given.)

How many milliliters will infuse per minute?

Find volume per minute.

Method: mL/min

Set up a ratio and proportion. Use volume/hour, 30 mL/hr, or 30 mL/60 min as the known variable.	30 mL : 60 min : : X mL : min 60 X = 30 X = 0.5 mL

Answer: The infusion rate for volume per minute is 0.5 mL/min and the hourly rate is 30 mL/hr.

What is the concentration per minute and hour?

Find concentration per minute.

Method: U/min

Multiply the concentration of solution by the volume per minute.	20 U/mL × 0.5 mL/min = 10 U/min

Find concentration per hour.

Method: U/hr

Multiply the volume per minute by 60 min/hr.	10 U/min × 60 min/hr = 600 U/hr

Answer: The concentration per minute of heparin is 10 U/min and the concentration per hour is 600 U/hr.

Concentration and Volume per Hour and Minute with a Drug in Milligrams

EXAMPLE

PROBLEM: Infuse lidocaine 2 g in D_5W 500 mL at 2 mg/min.

Concentration of solution is 4 mg/mL. (Also note that concentration/min is given.)

How many milligrams will be infused per hour?

Find concentration per hour.

Method: mg/hr

Find the concentration/minute. Multiply concentration/min × 60 min/hr.	lidocaine 2 mg/min 2 mg/min × 60 min = 120 mg/hr

Answer: The amount of lidocaine infused per hour is 120 mg/hr.

How many milliliters of lidocaine will infuse in 1 hour?
Find volume per hour.

Method: mL/hr

Calculate concentration of solution. Divide the concentration/hr by the concentration of solution.	lidocaine 4 mg/mL $\dfrac{120 \ \text{mg/hr}}{4 \ \text{mg/mL}} = 30 \ \text{mL/hr}$

Answer: The infusion rate in milliliters for lidocaine 2 mg/min is 30 mL/hr.

How many milliliters of lidocaine will infuse in 1 minute?
Find volume per minute.

Method: mL/min

Divide the concentration/min by the concentration of solution.	$\dfrac{2 \ \text{mg/min}}{4 \ \text{mg/mL}} = 0.5 \ \text{mL/min}$

Answer: The infusion rate for lidocaine 2 mg/min is 0.5 mL/min.

Concentration and Volume per Minute and Hour with a Drug in Micrograms

EXAMPLE

PROBLEM: Infuse dobutamine 250 mg in D_5W 500 mL at 650 mcg/min. Concentration of solution is 500 mcg/mL. Also note concentration/min is given in the order.

How many micrograms will infuse in 1 hour?

Find concentration per hour.

Method: mcg/hr

Find the concentration/min. Multiply concentration/min by 60 min/hr.	dobutamine 650 mcg/min $$650 \text{ mcg/min} \times 60 \text{ min/hr} = 39,000 \text{ mcg/hr}$$

Answer: The concentration of dobutamine infused per hour is 39,000 mcg/hr.

How many milliliters of dobutamine will infuse in 1 hour?

Find volume per hour.

Method: mL/hr

Calculate concentration of solution. Divide the concentration/hr by the concentration of solution.	dobutamine 500 mcg/mL $$\frac{39,000 \text{ mcg/hr}}{500 \text{ mcg/mL}} = 78 \text{ mL/hr}$$

Answer: The infusion rate for dobutamine 650 mcg/min is 78 mL/hr.

How many milliliters of dobutamine should infuse in 1 minute?

Find volume per minute.

Method: mL/min

Divide concentration/min by concentration of solution.	$$\frac{650 \text{ mcg/min}}{500 \text{ mcg/mL}} = 1.3 \text{ mL/min}$$

Answer: The infusion rate for dobutamine is 1.3 mL/min.

II. Practice Problems: Calculating Infusion Rate

Use the examples to find the following:

🖛 Concentration of the solution
🖛 Infusion rates per unit time

    a. Volume per minute
    b. Volume per hour
    c. Concentration per minute
    d. Concentration per hour

1. Order: heparin 1000 U in D_5W 500 mL at 50 mL/hr.

_____

2. Order: nitroprusside 100 mg in D_5W 500 mL at 60 mL/hr.

_____

3. Order: nitroprusside 25 mg in D_5W 250 mL at 50 mcg/min.

_____

4. Order: dopamine 800 mg in D_5W 500 mL at 400 mcg/min.

_____

5. Order: norepinephrine 2 mg in D_5W 250 mL at 45 mL/hr.

_____

6. Order: dobutamine 1000 mg in D_5W 500 mL at 12 mL/hr.

_____

7. Order: dobutamine 250 mg in D_5W 250 mL at 10 mL/hr.

_____

8. Order: lidocaine 2 g in D_5W 500 mL at 4 mg/min.

_____

9. Order: dopamine 400 mg in D_5W 250 mL at 60 mL/hr.

_____

10. Order: isoproterenol 4 mg in D_5W 500 mL at 65 mL/hr.

_____

11. Order: morphine sulfate 50 mg in 150 mL NSS at 3 mg/hr.

_____

12. Order: regular Humulin insulin 50 U in 250 mL NSS at 4 U/hr.

_____

13. Order: aminophylline 2 g in 250 mL D_5W at 20 mL/hr.

_____

14. Order: nitroglycerin 50 mg in 250 mL D₅W at 24 mL/hr.

_____

15. Order: heparin 25,000 U in 500 mL D₅W at 10 mL/hr.

_____

CALCULATING INFUSION RATES OF A DRUG FOR SPECIFIC BODY WEIGHT PER UNIT TIME

The last method is calculating infusion rates for the amount of drug per unit time for a specific body weight. The weight parameter is an accurate means of dosing for a therapeutic effect. The metric system is used for all drug dosing, so pounds must be changed to kilograms. The physician orders the _desired dose per kilogram of body weight_ and the _concentration of the solution._ From this information, infusion rates can be calculated for administering an individualized dose. Accurate daily weights are essential for the correct dosage.

The previous methods for calculating _concentration of solution_ and _infusion rates_ for concentration and volume are used, with one addition. The _concentration per minute_ is obtained by multiplying the _body weight_ by the _desired dose per kilogram per minute_ and must be done before calculating the other infusion rates. For many vasoactive drugs given as examples in this chapter, the most useful information clinically is the concentration per minute for the specific body weight, volume per minute, and volume per hour, because these determine the infusion pump settings.

Volumetric pumps do not infuse fractional portions of a milliliter, for example, 1.08 mL/hr. Therefore, if the volume per hour is a fractional amount, it must be rounded off to a whole number (1.8 mL/hr = 2 mL/hr). When calculating concentration per minute and hour and volume per minute, carry out the problem to three decimal places, if necessary, before rounding off. The volume per hour, if fractional, can then be rounded off, making the volume per hour as accurate as possible. There are two exceptions to rounding off fractional infusion rates. First, if the patient's condition is labile, the difference between 1 or 2 mL could be important. Secondly, since physicians order the medication, they must be consulted if rounding off would significantly change the drug dosage.

Micrograms per Kilogram Body Weight

EXAMPLE

PROBLEM: Infuse dobutamine 250 mg in 500 mL D₅W at 10 mcg/kg/min.

Patient weighs 143 lb.

Concentration of solution is 500 mcg/mL.

How many micrograms of dobutamine would infuse per minute? Per hour?

Convert pounds to kilograms.

Divide pounds by 2.2. $\dfrac{143 \; \cancel{lb}}{2.2 \; \cancel{lb}/kg} = kg$

Find concentration per minute.

Method: mcg/min

Multiply patient's weight by the desired dose of mcg/kg/min.	65 kg × 10 mcg/kg/min = 650 mcg/min

Find concentration per hour.

Method: mcg/hr

Multiply concentration/min by 60 min/hr.	650 mcg/min × 60 min/hr = 39,000 mcg/hr

Answer: The concentration of dobutamine infused per minute and hour is 650 mcg/min and 39,000 mcg/hr for the patient's body weight.

How many milliliters of dobutamine will infuse per minute? Per hour?

Find volume per minute.

Method: mL/min

Divide the concentration/min by the concentration of the solution.	$\dfrac{650 \; \cancel{mcg}/min}{500 \; \cancel{mcg}/mL} = 1.241 \; mL/min$

Find volume per hour.

Method: mL/hr

Multiply volume/min by 60 min/hr.	1.241 mL/min × 60 min/hr = 74.46 or 74 mL/hr

Answer: The volume of dobutamine infused per minute is 1.241 mL/min, and the infusion rate per hour is 74 mL/hr.

BASIC FRACTIONAL FORMULA

A fractional equation can create a basic formula that can be used as another quick method to determine any one of the following quantities: concentration of solution, volume per hour, or desired concentration per minute ($\times$ kilogram of body weight, if required). The equation has one constant, the drop rate of the IV set, 60 gtt/mL. The unknown quantity can be represented by X. (See Chap. 3 for fractional equations.) The basic formula is not accurate to the nearest hundredth, as are the other methods in this section.

$$\frac{\text{concentration of solution (U, mg, mcg/mL)}}{\text{drop rate of set (60 gtt/mL)}}$$

$$= \frac{\text{desired concentration/min} \times \text{kg body weight}}{\text{volume/hr (mL/hr or gtt/min)}}$$

1. Use the formula to find the volume per hour or drops per minute.

EXAMPLE

Infuse heparin 5000 U in 250 mL D_5W at 0.15 U/kg/min. Patient weighs 70 kg. The concentration of solution is 20 U/mL.

Desired concentration/minute: 0.15 U/kg/min $\times$ 70 kg = 10.5 U/min

$$\frac{20 \text{ U/mL}}{60 \text{ gtt/mL}} = \frac{10.5 \text{ U/min}}{\text{X (mL/hr or gtt/min)}}$$

$$20 \text{ X} = 630$$

$$\text{X} = 31 \text{ mL/hr or 31 gtt/min}$$

2. Use the formula to find the desired concentration per minute.

EXAMPLE

Infuse lidocaine 2 g in 500 mL D_5W at 30 mL/hr. The concentration of solution is 4 mg/mL.

$$\frac{4 \text{ mg/mL}}{60 \text{ gtt/mL}} = \frac{\text{X}}{30 \text{ mL/hr}}$$

$$60 \text{ X} = 120$$
$$\text{X} = 2 \text{ mg/min}$$

3. Use the formula to find the concentration of solution.

EXAMPLE

Infuse dobutamine 250 mg in D_5W 500 mL at 10 mcg/kg/min with rate of 74 mL/hr. Patient weighs 65 kg.

Desired concentration per minute = 10 mcg/kg/min $\times$ 65 kg
= 650 mcg/min

$$\frac{\text{X}}{60 \text{ gtt/mL}} = \frac{650 \text{ mcg/min}}{78 \text{ mL/hr}}$$

$$74 \text{ X} = 39,000$$
$$\text{X} = 527 \text{ mcg/mL}$$

III. Practice Problems: Calculating Infusion Rate for Specific Body Weight

Determine the infusion rates for specific body weight by calculating the following.

🖋 Concentration of the solution
🖋 Weight in kilograms
🖋 Infusion rates
    a. Concentration per minute
    b. Concentration per hour (not always measured)
    c. Volume per minute
    d. Volume per hour

You can use the basic fractional formula and compare answers.

1. Infuse dobutamine 500 mg in 250 mL D$_5$W at 5 mcg/kg/min. Patient weighs 182 lb.

___

2. Infuse amrinone 250 mg in 250 mL NSS at 5 mcg/kg/min. Patient weighs 165 lb.

___

3. Infuse dopamine 400 mg in 250 mL D$_5$W at 10 mcg/kg/min. Patient weighs 140 lb.

___

4. Infuse nitroprusside 100 mg in 500 mL D$_5$W at 3 mcg/kg/min. Patient weighs 55 kg.

___

5. Infuse dobutamine 1000 mg in 500 mL D$_5$W at 15 mcg/kg/min. Patient weighs 110 lb.

___

TITRATION OF INFUSION RATE

Drugs administered by titration are based on *concentration of solution, infusion rates, specific concentration per kilogram of body weight,* and *titration factor.* The titration factor is the concentration of drug per drop in U/gtt, mg/gtt, or mcg/gtt. The titration factor can be added to or subtracted from the baseline infusion rate to determine the exact concentration of an infusion. Because the titration method of drug administration is primarily used when a patient's condition is labile, calculating the titration factor will give the nurse the means for determining the exact amount of drug being infused.

Charts for drug infusion, developed by drug manufacturers, can be used for adjusting infusion rates for drug titrations. Often, the amount of drug being infused falls between calibrations on the charts. When this occurs, the titration factor can be used to determine the exact concentration of drug being administered. The titration factor can also be used to verify the correct selection from the chart.

EXAMPLE

Infuse Isuprel 2 mg in 250 mL D_5W.

Titrate 1–3 mcg/min to maintain heart rate > 50 and < 130 and blood pressure > 90 systolic.

a. Concentration of solution

Convert mg to mcg. Set up ratio and proportion.	2 mg = 2000 mcg 2000 mcg : 250 mL : : X mcg : mL 250 X = 2000 X = 8 mcg 8 mcg/mL

b. Infusion rate by volume per unit time

Desired infusion rate by concentration is stated in the problem. Note that the upper dosage and lower dosage must be determined.

REMEMBER: Hourly rate and the number of drops per minute are the same with a microdrip administration set.

VOLUME RATE PER MINUTE: mL/min

	Lower	Upper
Divide concentration/min by concentration of solution.	$\dfrac{1 \text{ mcg/min}}{8 \text{ mcg/mL}}$	$\dfrac{3 \text{ mcg/min}}{8 \text{ mcg/mL}}$
	= 0.125 mL/min	= 0.375 mL/min

VOLUME RATE PER HOUR: mL/hr (equivalent to gtt/min)

	Lower
Multiply volume rate/min by 60 min.	0.125 mL/min × 60 min/hr = 7.5 mL/hr (7.5 gtt/min)

Upper

0.375 mL/hr × 60 min/hr
= 22.5 mL/hr (22.5 gtt/min)

c. Titration factor

Find rate in gtt/min. Divide concentration/min by gtt/min.	7.5 gtt/min $\dfrac{1 \text{ mcg/min}}{7.5 \text{ gtt/min}} = 0.133 \text{ mcg/gt}$

The *titration factor* is 0.133 mcg/gtt in a solution of Isuprel 2 mg in 250 mL D$_5$W. To repeat, changing drops per minute results in a corresponding change in milliliters per hour. If the baseline infusion rates are **1 mcg/min** for concentration and **7.5 mL/hr** for volume, increasing the infusion rate by **1 gt/min** changes the concentration/minute by **0.133 mcg** and increases the hourly volume by **1 mL** to give a rate of **8.5 mL/hr.**

d. Increasing or decreasing rates

To increase the infusion rate by 5 gtt/min from a baseline rate of 1 mcg/min, set up a ratio and proportion or multiply the titration factor (mcg/gtt) by 5 to obtain the increment of increase.

E X A M P L E

Set up a ratio and proportion with rate in gtt/min as the known variables.

7.5 gtt : 1 mcg : : 5 gtt : X mcg
7.5 X = 5
X = 0.666 mcg
5 gtt/0.66 mcg

or

Multiply titration factor in mcg/gtt by 5.

0.133 mcg/gtt × 5 gtt
= 0.665 mcg

By adding 5 gtt/min, the volume infusion rate has increased 5 mL/hr from 7.5 to 12.5 mL/hr. The concentration of drug delivered is increased by 0.665 mcg/min to 1.665 mcg/min. For example,

$$
\begin{array}{ll}
1.000 \text{ mcg/min} & \text{baseline rate} \\
+ \; \underline{0.665} \text{ mcg/min} & \text{increment of rate increased} \\
1.665 \text{ mcg/min} & \text{adjusted infusion rate}
\end{array}
$$

Suppose the infusion rate was 3 mcg/min and a decrease was needed. To decrease the infusion rate by 10 gtt, set up another ratio and proportion or multiply the titration factor (mcg/gtt) by 10.

E X A M P L E

Set up a ratio and proportion with rate in gtt/mcg as the known variable.

7.5 gtt : 1 mcg : : 10 gtt : X mcg
7.5 X = 10
X = 1.33 mcg
1.33 mcg/10 gtt

or

Multiply titration factor in
mcg/gtt by 10.

0.133 mcg/gtt × 10 gtt
= 1.33 mcg

By subtracting 10 gtt/min, the infusion rate has decreased 10 mL/hr from 22.5 to 12.5 mL/hr. The amount of drug delivered is decreased by 1.33 mcg/min to 1.67 mcg/min. For example,

$$
\begin{array}{ll}
3.00 \text{ mcg/min} & \text{baseline infusion rate} \\
- \underline{1.33} \text{ mcg/min} & \text{increment of rate decreased} \\
1.67 \text{ mcg/min} & \text{adjusted infusion rate}
\end{array}
$$

IV. Practice Problems: Titration of Infusion Rate

1. What are the units of measure for the following terms?
   a. Concentration of solution per minute for specific body weight

   _____

   b. Concentration of solution

   _____

   c. Volume per hour

   _____

   d. Concentration per minute

   _____

   e. Volume per minute

   _____

   f. Concentration per minute

   _____

2. Order: nitroprusside 50 mg in 250 mL D₅W. Titrate 0.5–1.5 mcg/kg/min to maintain mean systolic blood pressure at 100 mm Hg. Patient weighs 70 kg.
   Find the following:
   a. Concentration of solution

   _____

   b. Concentration per minute

   _____

   c. Volume per minute and hour

   _____

   d. Titration factor

   _____

e. Increase the infusion rate of 11 gtt/min by 5 gtt. What is the concentration per minute? What is the volume per hour?

_____

f. Increase the infusion rate of 16 gtt/mL by 13 gtt. What is the concentration per minute? What is the volume per hour?

_____

3. Order: dopamine 400 mg in 250 mL D$_5$W. Titrate beginning at 4 mcg/kg/min to maintain a mean systolic blood pressure of 100 to 120 mm Hg. Patient weighs 75 kg.

Find the following:

a. Concentration of solution

_____

b. Concentration per minute

_____

c. Volume per minute and hour

_____

d. Titration factor

_____

e. Increase the infusion rate of 113 gtt/min by 7 gtt. What is the concentration per minute? What is the volume per hour?

_____

f. Decrease the infusion rate of 120 mL/hr (120 gtt/min) by 5 gtt. What is the concentration per minute? What is the volume per hour?

_____

"FACTOR OF 15" METHOD

The "factor of 15" method is another means to prepare vasoactive drugs, particularly those given in micrograms per kilogram of body weight per minute (mcg/kg/min). The advantages of this method are that the dosage of vasoactive drug is delivered in a higher concentration with less volume and that the dose is highly individualized. This method is useful in patients with cardiac and renal disorders when fluids must be restricted.

The amount of drug is determined by multiplying the patient's weight in kilograms by 15; when the drug is mixed in 250 mL of IV fluid, the solution will always have a concentration of 1 mcg/kg/min. The formula used to derive the conversion factor is

$$\frac{(1 \text{ mcg/kg/gtt})(60 \text{ gtt/mL})(250 \text{ mL})(\text{kg body weight})}{1000 \text{ mcg/mg}} = X \text{ mg of drug}$$

$$15 \times \text{kg body weight} = X \text{ mg of drug}$$

EXAMPLE

Order: dobutamine 20 mcg/min. Patient weighs 60 kg.

$$\frac{(1 \text{ mcg/kg/gtt})(60 \text{ gtt/mL})(250 \text{ mL})(60 \text{ kg})}{1000 \text{ mcg/mg}} = X \text{ mg of drug}$$

$$15 \times 60 \text{ kg} = 900 \text{ mg of drug}$$

900 mg of dobutamine in 250 mL D_5W will yield a concentration of 1 mcg/kg/min.

When using this method, the physician should include the exact amount of drug needed in the order. For example,

Mix 900 mg dobutamine in 250 mL D_5W and infuse at 20 mcg/min.

The limitation of the ''factor of 15'' method is that it cannot be used for all vasoactive drugs. If the drug is manufactured in a very small concentration (in a small volume such as 1 mg/mL), too many vials would be used to mix the correct concentration. If a very large concentration of drug were mixed in a small volume such as 1000 mg in 5 mL, it would be very difficult to accurately draw up the amount with a syringe. In addition, other safety measures must be taken with this method. One is using a pump or controller to make sure the patient does not receive any extra fluid or drug. Another is placing a stopcock in the IV line between the patient and the pump or controller so that air can be removed without the patient getting extra medication. All patients on vasoactive drugs should be monitored invasively to obtain the most accurate data for treatment.

V. Practice Problems: "Factor of 15" Method

1. Dopamine is to be administered at 10 mcg/min. The patient weighs 74 kg. According to the ''factor of 15'' method, how much dopamine should be added to 250 mL of D_5W?
2. Dobutamine is to be given at 15 mcg/min. The patient weighs 80 kg. According to the ''factor of 15'' method, how much dobutamine should be added to 250 mL D_5W?

TOTAL AMOUNT OF DRUG INFUSED OVER TIME

Determining the total amount of drug infused over time is useful when changes in drug therapy occur. If adverse effects, toxic levels, therapeutic failure, or discontinuance of a drug occurs, knowing the amount that was administered can be important for charting and for determining future therapies.

For this calculation, the concentration of the drug in solution must be known, as must the time that drug therapy began to the nearest minute. Again, with 60-gtt sets, the hourly rate is the same as the drip rate per minute.

EXAMPLE

Heparin 10,000 U in 250 mL D$_5$W at 30 mL/hr has been infusing for 3 hours. The drug is discontinued.

How much heparin did the patient receive?

Concentration of solution

Set up a ratio and proportion.	10,000 U : 250 mL : : X U : mL
Solve for X.	250 X = 10,000
	X = 40 U
	40 U/mL

Concentration per hour

| Multiply concentration of solution by volume/hr. | 40 U/mL × 30 mL/hr = 1200 U/hr |

Total amount of drug infused

| Multiply concentration/hr by length of administration. | 1200 U/hr × 3 hr = 3600 U/3 hr |

Answer: The total amount of heparin that infused over 3 hours was 3600 U.

| **VI. Practice Problems: Total Amount of Drug Infused Over Time** |

Solve for the amount of drug infused over time.

1. In 1 hour, a patient received two boluses of lidocaine 100 mg and an IV infusion of 4 mg/mL at 40 mL/hr for 30 min. How many milligrams have infused?

Note: Do not exceed 300 mg/hr of lidocaine.

2. Heparin 20,000 U in 500 mL D$_5$W at 50 mL/hr has been infusing for · 5½ hours. The drug is discontinued. How much heparin has been given?

ANSWERS

I. Calculating Concentration of a Solution

1. 10,000 U : 250 mL : : X U : mL
   250 X = 10,000
   X = 40 U

   The concentration of solution is 40 U/mL.

2. 250 mg : 500 mL : : X mg : mL
500 X = 250
X = 0.5 mg

The concentration of solution is 0.5 mg/mL.

3. 100 U : 500 mL : : X U : mL
500 X = 100
X = 0.2 U

The concentration of solution is 0.2 U/mL.

4. 1 g = 1000 mg
1000 mg : 1000 mL : : X mg : mL
1000 X = 1000
X = 1 mg

The concentration of solution is 1 mg/mL.

5. 4 mg = 4000 mcg
4000 mcg : 500 mL : : X mcg : mL
500 X = 4000
X = 8 mcg

The concentration of solution is 8 mcg/mL.

6. 500 mg : 250 mL : : X mcg : mL
250 X = 500
X = 2 mg

The concentration of solution is 2 mg/mL.

7. 400 mg : 250 mL : : X mg : mL
250 X = 400
X = 1.6 mg

The concentration of solution is 1.6 mg/mL.

8. 2 mg = 2000 mcg
2000 mcg : 250 mL : : X mcg : mL
250 X = 2000
X = 8 mcg

The concentration of solution is 8 mcg/mL.

9. 750,000 U : 50 mL : : X U : mL
50 X = 750,000
X = 15,000 U

The concentration of solution is 15,000 U/mL.

10. 50 mg = 50,000 mcg
50,000 mcg : 500 mL : : X mcg : mL
500 X = 50,000
X = 100 mcg

The concentration of solution is 100 mcg/mL.

11. 1 g = 1000 mg
1000 mg : 250 mL : : X mg : mL
250 X = 1000
X = 4 mg

The concentration of solution is 4 mg/mL.

12. 2 g = 2000 mg
2000 mg : 250 mL : : X mg : mL
250 X = 2000
X = 8 mg

The concentration of solution is 8 mg/mL.

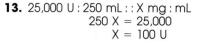
13. 25,000 U : 250 mL : : X mg : mL
250 X = 25,000
X = 100 U

The concentration of solution is 100 U/mL.

14.   1 g = 1000 mg
1000 mg : 500 mL : : X mg : mL
500 X = 1000
X = 2 mg

The concentration of solution is 2 mg/mL.

15.   50 mg = 50,000 mcg
50,000 mcg : 250 mL : : X mcg : mL
250 X = 50,000 mcg
X = 200 mcg

The concentration of solution is 200 mcg/mL.

II. Calculating Infusion Rate

1. *Concentration of solution*

1000 U : 500 mL = X U : mL
500 X = 1000
X = 2 U

The concentration of solution is 2 U/mL.

Infusion rates

a. Volume/min

50 mL : 60 min : : X mL : min
60 X = 50
X = 0.833 mL or 0.83 mL
0.83 mL/min

b. Volume/hr

50 mL/hr

c. Concentration/min

2 U/mL × 0.83 mL/min = 1.66 U/min

d. Concentration/hr

1.66 U/min × 60 min/hr = 99.6 U/hr or 100 U/hr

2. *Concentration of solution*

100 mg : 500 mL : : X mg : mL
500 X = 100
X = 0.2 mg

The concentration of solution is 0.2 mg/mL.

Infusion rates

a. Volume/min

60 mL : 60 min : : X mL : min
60 X = 60
X = 1 mL
1 mL/min

b. Volume/hr

60 mL/hr

c. Concentration/min

0.2 mg/mL × 1 mL/min = 0.2 mg/min

d. Concentration/hr

0.2 mg/min × 60 min/hr = 12 mg/hr

3. *Concentration of solution*

$$25 \text{ mg} = 25,000 \text{ mcg}$$
$$25,000 \text{ mcg} : 250 \text{ mL} :: X \text{ mcg} : \text{mL}$$
$$250 X = 25,000$$
$$X = 100 \text{ mcg}$$

The concentration of solution is 100 mcg/ml.

Infusion rates

a. Volume/min

$$\frac{50 \text{ mcg/min}}{100 \text{ mcg/mL}} = 0.5 \text{ mL/min}$$

b. Volume/hr

$$0.5 \text{ mL/min} \times 60 \text{ min/hr} = 30 \text{ mL/hr}$$

c. Concentration/min

$$50 \text{ mcg/min}$$

d. Concentration/hr

$$50 \text{ mcg/min} \times 60 \text{ min/hr} = 3000 \text{ mcg/hr}$$

4. *Concentration of solution*

$$800 \text{ mg} = 800,000 \text{ mcg}$$
$$800,000 \text{ mcg} : 500 \text{ mL} :: X \text{ mcg} : \text{mL}$$
$$500 X = 800,000$$
$$X = 1600 \text{ mcg}$$

The concentration of solution is 1600 mcg/mL.

Infusion rates

a. Volume/min

$$\frac{400 \text{ mcg/min}}{1600 \text{ mcg/mL}} = 0.25 \text{ mL/min}$$

b. Volume/hr

$$0.25 \text{ mL/min} \times 60 \text{ min/hr} = 15 \text{ mL/hr}$$

c. Concentration/min

$$400 \text{ mcg/min}$$

d. Concentration/hr

$$400 \text{ mcg/min} \times 60 \text{ min/hr} = 24,000 \text{ mcg/hr}$$

5. *Concentration of solution*

$$2 \text{ mg} = 2000 \text{ mcg}$$
$$2000 \text{ mcg} : 250 \text{ mL} :: X \text{ mcg} : \text{mL}$$
$$250 X = 2000$$
$$X = 8 \text{ mcg}$$

The concentration of solution is 8 mcg/mL.

Infusion rates

a. Volume/min

$$45 \text{ mL} : 60 \text{ min} :: X \text{ mL} : \text{min}$$
$$60 X = 45$$
$$X = 0.75 \text{ mL/min}$$

b. Volume/hr

$$45 \text{ mL/hr}$$

c. Concentration/min

$$8 \text{ mcg/mL} \times 0.75 \text{ mL/min} = 6 \text{ mcg/min}$$

d. Concentration/hr

$$6 \text{ mcg/min} \times 60 \text{ min/hr} = 360 \text{ mcg/hr}$$

6. *Concentration of solution*

$$1000 \text{ mg} = 1,000,000 \text{ mcg}$$
$$1,000,000 \text{ mcg} : 500 \text{ mL} :: X \text{ mcg} : \text{mL}$$
$$500 X = 1,000,000$$
$$X = 2000 \text{ mcg}$$

The concentration of solution is 2000 mcg/mL.

Infusion rates

a. Volume/min

$$12 \text{ mL} : 60 \text{ min} :: X \text{ mL} : \text{min}$$
$$60 X = 12$$
$$X = 0.2 \text{ mL}$$
$$0.2 \text{ mL/min}$$

b. Volume/hr

$$12 \text{ mL/hr}$$

c. Concentration/min

$$2000 \text{ mcg/mL} \times 0.2 \text{ mL/min} = 400 \text{ mcg/min}$$

d. Concentration/hr

$$400 \text{ mcg/min} \times 60 \text{ min/hr} = 24,000 \text{ mcg/hr7}$$

7. *Concentration of solution*

$$250 \text{ mg} = 250,000 \text{ mcg}$$
$$250,000 \text{ mcg} : 250 \text{ mL} :: X \text{ mcg} : \text{mL}$$
$$250 X = 250,000$$
$$X = 1000 \text{ mcg}$$

The concentration of solution is 1000 mcg/mL.

Infusion rates

a. Volume/min

$$10 \text{ mL} : 60 \text{ min} :: X \text{ mL} : 1 \text{ min}$$
$$60 X = 10 \text{ mL}$$
$$X = 0.1666 \text{ mL or } 0.167 \text{ mL}$$
$$0.167 \text{ mL/min}$$

b. Volume/hr

$$10 \text{ mL/hr}$$

c. Concentration/min

$$1000 \text{ mcg/mL} \times 0.167 \text{ mL/min} = 167 \text{ mcg/min}$$

d. Concentration/hr

$$167 \text{ mcg/min} \times 60 \text{ min/hr} = 10,020 \text{ mcg/hr or } 10,000 \text{ mcg/hr}$$

8. *Concentration of solution*

$$2 \text{ g} = 2000 \text{ mg}$$
$$2000 \text{ mg} : 500 \text{ mL} :: X \text{ mg} : \text{mL}$$
$$500 X = 2000$$
$$X = 4 \text{ mg}$$

The concentration of solution is 4 mg/mL.

Infusion rates

a. Volume/min

$$\frac{4 \text{ mg/mL}}{4 \text{ mg/min}} = 1 \text{ mL/min}$$

b. Volume/hr

$$1 \text{ mL/min} \times 60 \text{ min/hr} = 60 \text{ mL/hr}$$

c. Concentration/min

$$4 \text{ mg/min}$$

d. Concentration/hr

$$4 \text{ mg/min} \times 60 \text{ min/hr} = 240 \text{ mg/hr}$$

9. *Concentration of solution*

$$400 \text{ mg} : 250 \text{ mL} :: X \text{ mg} : \text{mL}$$
$$250 X = 400$$
$$X = 1.6 \text{ mg}$$

The concentration of solution is 1.6 mg/mL.

Infusion rates

a. Volume/min

$$60 \text{ mL} : 60 \text{ min} :: X \text{ mL} : \text{min}$$
$$60 X = 60$$
$$X = 1 \text{ mL}$$
$$1 \text{ mL/min}$$

b. Volume/hr

$$60 \text{ mL/hr}$$

c. Concentration/min

$$1.6 \text{ mg/mL} \times 1 \text{ mL/min} = 1.6 \text{ mg/min}$$

d. Concentration/hr

$$1.6 \text{ mg/min} \times 60 \text{ min/hr} = 96 \text{ mg/hr}$$

10. *Concentration of solution*

$$4 \text{ mg} = 4000 \text{ mcg}$$
$$4000 \text{ mcg} : 500 \text{ mL} :: X \text{ mcg} : \text{mL}$$
$$500 X = 4000$$
$$X = 8 \text{ mcg}$$

The concentration of solution is 8 mcg/mL.

Infusion rates

a. Volume/min

$$65 \text{ mL} : 60 \text{ min} :: X \text{ mL} : \text{min}$$
$$60 X = 65$$
$$X = 1.083 \text{ mL}$$
$$1.08 \text{ mL/min}$$

b. Volume/hr

$$65 \text{ mL/hr}$$

c. Concentration/min

$$8 \text{ mcg/mL} \times 1.08 \text{ mL/min} = 8.64 \text{ mcg/min}$$

d. Concentration/hr

$$8.64 \text{ mcg/min} \times 60 \text{ min/hr} = 518.4 \text{ mcg/hr}$$

11. *Concentration of solution*

$$50 \text{ mg} : 150 \text{ mL} :: X \text{ mg} : \text{mL}$$
$$150 X = 50$$
$$X = 0.33 \text{ mg}$$

The concentration of solution is 0.33 mg/mL.

Infusion rates

a. Concentration/min

$$3 \text{ mg} : 60 \text{ min} :: X \text{ mg} : \text{min}$$
$$60 X = 3$$
$$X = 0.05 \text{ mg/min}$$

b. Concentration/hr

$$3 \text{ mg/hr}$$

c. Volume/min

$$\frac{0.05 \text{ mg/min}}{0.33 \text{ mg/mL}} = 0.15 \text{ mL/min}$$

d. Volume/hr

$$\frac{3 \text{ mg/hr}}{0.33 \text{ mg/mL}} = 9.09 \text{ or } 9 \text{ mL/hr}$$

12. *Concentration of solution*

$$50 \text{ U} : 250 \text{ mL} : : X \text{ mg} : \text{mL}$$
$$250 \text{ X} = 50$$
$$X = 0.2 \text{ U}$$

The concentration of solution is 0.2 U/mL.

Infusion rates

a. Concentration/min

$$4 \text{ U} : 60 \text{ min} : : X \text{ U} : \text{min}$$
$$60 \text{ X} = 4$$
$$X = 0.066 \text{ U/min}$$

b. Concentration/hr

$$4 \text{ U/hr}$$

c. Volume/min

$$\frac{0.66 \text{ U/min}}{0.2 \text{ U/mL}} = 0.33 \text{ mL/min}$$

d. Volume/hr

$$\frac{4 \text{ U/hr}}{0.2 \text{ U/mL}} = 20 \text{ mL/hr}$$

13. *Concentration of solution*

$$2 \text{ g} = 2000 \text{ mg}$$
$$2000 \text{ mg} : 250 \text{ mL} : : X \text{ mg} : \text{mL}$$
$$250 \text{ X} = 2000$$
$$X = 8 \text{ mg}$$

The concentration of solution is 8 mg/mL.

Infusion rates

a. Volume/hr = 20 mL/hr

b. Volume/min

$$20 \text{ mL} : 60 \text{ min/hr} : : X \text{ mL} : \text{min}$$
$$60 \text{ X} = 20$$
$$X = 0.3 \text{ mL/min}$$

c. Concentration/min

$$8 \text{ mg/mL} \times 0.3 \text{ mL/min} = 2.4 \text{ mg/min}$$

d. Concentration/hr

$$2.4 \text{ mg/min} \times 60 \text{ min/hr} = 360 \text{ mg/hr}$$

14. *Concentration of solution*

$$50 \text{ mg} = 50,000 \text{ mcg}$$
$$50,000 \text{ mcg} : 250 \text{ mL} : : X \text{ mg} : \text{mL}$$
$$250 \text{ X} = 50,000$$
$$X = 200 \text{ mcg}$$

The concentration of solution is 200 mcg/mL.

Infusion rates

a. Volume/hr = 24 mL/hr

b. Volume/min

$$24 \text{ mL/hr} : 60 \text{ min/hr} :: X \text{ mL} : \text{min}$$
$$60 \text{ X} = 24$$
$$X = 0.4 \text{ mL/min}$$

c. Concentration/min

$$200 \text{ mcg/mL} \times 0.4 \text{ mL/min} = 80 \text{ mcg/min}$$

d. Concentration/hr

$$80 \text{ mcg/min} \times 60 \text{ min} = 4800 \text{ mcg/hr}$$

15. *Concentration of solution*

$$25,000 \text{ U} : 500 \text{ mL} :: X \text{ U} : \text{mL}$$
$$500 \text{ X} = 25,000$$
$$X = 50 \text{ U}$$

The concentration of solution is 50 U/mL.

Infusion rates

a. Volume/hr

$$10 \text{ mL/hr}$$

b. Volume/min

$$10 \text{ mL} : 60 \text{ min/hr} :: X \text{ mL} : \text{min}$$
$$60 \text{ X} = 10$$
$$X = 0.165 \text{ mL/min}$$

c. Concentration/hr

$$50 \text{ U/mL} \times 10 \text{ mL/hr} = 500 \text{ U/hr}$$

d. Concentration/min

$$50 \text{ U/mL} \times 0.165 \text{ mL/min} = 8.25 \text{ U/min}$$

III. Calculating Infusion Rate for Specific Body Weight

1. *Concentration of solution*   *lb to kg*

$$500 \text{ mg} = 500,000 \text{ mcg} \qquad \frac{182}{2.2} = 82.7 \text{ kg}$$
$$500,000 : 250 \text{ mL} :: X \text{ mcg} : \text{mL}$$
$$250 \text{ X} = 500,000$$
$$X = 2000 \text{ mcg}$$

The concentration of solution is 2000 mcg/mL.

Infusion rates

a. Concentration/min

$$\text{body weight} \times \text{desired dose/kg/min}$$
$$82.7 \text{ kg} \times 5 \text{ mcg/kg/min}$$
$$= 413.4 \text{ mcg/min}$$

b. Concentration/hr

$$413.5 \text{ mcg/min} \times 60 \text{ min/hr} = 24,810 \text{ mcg/hr}$$

c. Volume/min

$$\frac{413.5 \text{ mcg/min}}{2000 \text{ mcg/mL}} = 0.206 \text{ mL/min}$$

d. Volume/hr

$$0.206 \text{ mL/min} \times 60 \text{ min/hr} = 12.36 \text{ or } 12 \text{ mL/hr}$$

2. *Concentration of solution*   *lb to kg*

$$250 \text{ mg} = 250{,}000 \text{ mcg}$$
$$250{,}000 \text{ mcg} : 250 \text{ mL} :: X \text{ mcg} : \text{mL}$$
$$250 \, X = 250{,}000$$
$$X = 1000 \text{ mcg}$$

$$\frac{165}{2.2} = 75 \text{ kg}$$

The concentration of solution is 1000 mcg/mL.

Infusion rates

a. Concentration/min

$$\text{body weight} \times \text{desired dose/kg/min}$$
$$75 \text{ kg} \times 5 \text{ mcg/kg/min} = 375 \text{ mcg/min}$$

b. Concentration/hr

$$375 \text{ mcg/min} \times 60 \text{ min/hr} = 22{,}500 \text{ mcg/hr}$$

c. Volume/min

$$\frac{375 \text{ mcg/min}}{1000 \text{ mcg/mL}} = 0.375 \text{ mL/min}$$

d. Volume/hr

$$0.375 \text{ mL/min} \times 60 \text{ min/hr} = 22.5 \text{ mL/hr or } 23 \text{ mL/hr}$$

3. *Concentration of solution*   *lb to kg*

$$400 \text{ mg} = 400{,}000 \text{ mcg}$$
$$400{,}000 \text{ mg} : 250 \text{ mL} :: X \text{ mg} : \text{mL}$$
$$250 \, X = 400{,}000$$
$$X = 1600 \text{ mcg}$$

$$\frac{140}{2.2} = 63.6 \text{ kg}$$

The concentration of solution is 1600 mcg/mL.

Infusion rates

a. Concentration/min

$$\text{body weight} \times \text{desired dose/kg/min}$$
$$63.6 \text{ kg} \times 10 \text{ mcg/kg/min}$$
$$= 636 \text{ mcg/min}$$

b. Concentration/hr

$$636 \text{ mcg/min} \times 60 \text{ min/hr} = 38{,}160 \text{ mcg/hr}$$

c. Volume/min

$$\frac{636 \text{ mcg/min}}{1600 \text{ mcg/mL}} = 0.39 \text{ mL/min}$$

d. Volume/hr

$$0.39 \text{ mL/min} \times 60 \text{ min/hr} = 23.4 \text{ mL/hr or } 23 \text{ mL/hr}$$

4. *Concentration of solution*   *Patient weight*

$$100 \text{ mg} = 100{,}000 \text{ mcg}$$
$$100{,}000 \text{ mcg} : 500 \text{ mL} :: X \text{ mg} : \text{mL}$$
$$500 \, X = 100{,}000$$
$$X = 200 \text{ mcg}$$

55 kg

The concentration of solution is 200 mcg/mL.

Infusion rates

a. Concentration/min

$$3 \text{ mcg/kg/min} \times 55 \text{ kg} = 165 \text{ mcg/min}$$

b. Concentration/hr

$$165 \text{ mcg/min} \times 60 \text{ min/hr} = 9900 \text{ mcg/hr}$$

c. Volume/min

$$\frac{165 \text{ mcg/min}}{200 \text{ mcg/mL}} = 0.825 \text{ mL/min}$$

d. Volume/hr

0.825 mL/min × 60 min/hr = 49.5 mL/hr or 50 mL/hr

5. *Concentration of solution*   *lb to kg*

$$1000 \text{ mg} = 1{,}000{,}000 \text{ mcg} \qquad \frac{110}{2.2} = 50 \text{ kg}$$

1,000,000 mcg : 500 mL : : X mcg : mL
500 X = 1,000,000
X = 2000 mcg

The concentration of solution is 2000 mcg/mL.

Infusion rates

a. Concentration/min

body weight × desired dose/kg/min
50 kg × 15 mcg/kg/min
= 750 mcg/min

b. Concentration/hr

750 mcg/min × 60 min/hr = 45,000 mcg/hr

c. Volume/min

$$\frac{750 \text{ mcg/min}}{2000 \text{ mcg/mL}} = 0.375 \text{ mL/min}$$

d. Volume/hr

0.375 mL/min × 60 min/hr = 22.5 mL/hr or 23 mL/hr

IV. Titration of Infusion Rate

1. a. (U, mg, mcg)/kg/min
  b. (U, mg, mcg)/mL
  c. mL/hr
  d. (U, mg, mcg)/min
  e. mL/min
  f. (U, mg, mcg)/min

2. a. Concentration of solution

50 mg = 50,000 mcg
50,000 mcg : 250 mL : : X mcg : 1 mL
250 X = 50,000
X = 200 mcg

The concentration of solution is 200 mcg/mL.

  b. Concentration/min

Lower: 0.5 mcg/kg/min × 70 kg = 35 mcg/min
Upper: 1.5 mcg/kg/min × 70 kg = 105 mcg/min

  c. Volume/min and hr

Lower: $\dfrac{35 \text{ mcg/min}}{200 \text{ mcg/mL}} = 0.175$ mL/min × 60 min/hr = 10.5 or 11 mL/hr

Upper: $\dfrac{105 \text{ mcg/min}}{200 \text{ mcg/mL}} = 0.525$ mL/min × 60 min/hr = 31.5 or 32 mL/hr

  d. Titration factor

11 mL/hr = 11 gtt/min $\dfrac{35 \text{ mcg/min}}{11 \text{ gtt/min}} = 3.18$ or 3 mcg/gtt

e.
$$5 \text{ gtt} \times 3 \text{ mcg/gtt} = 15 \text{ mcg}$$
$$15 \text{ mcg} + 35 \text{ mcg/min} = 50 \text{ mcg/min}$$
$$5 \text{ gtt} + 11 \text{ gtt/min} = 16 \text{ gtt/min or } 16 \text{ mL/hr}$$

f. $13 \text{ gtt} \times 3 \text{ mcg/gtt} = 39 \text{ mcg}$ $39 \text{ mcg} + 50 \text{ mcg} = 89 \text{ mcg/min}$
$$13 \text{ gtt} + 16 \text{ gtt} = 29 \text{ gtt/mL or } 29 \text{ mL/hr}$$

3. a. Concentration of solution
$$400 \text{ mg} = 40,000 \text{ mcg}$$
$$40,000 \text{ mcg} : 250 \text{ mL} : : X \text{ mcg} : 1 \text{ mL}$$
$$250 \text{ X} = 40,000 \text{ mcg}$$
$$X = 160 \text{ mcg}$$

The concentration of solution is 160 mcg/mL.

b. Concentration/min
$$4 \text{ mcg/kg/min} \times 75 \text{ kg} = 300 \text{ mcg/min}$$

c. Volume/min and hr
$$\frac{300 \text{ mcg/min}}{160 \text{ mcg/mL}} = 1.875 \text{ mL/min} \times 60 \text{ min/hr} = 112.5 \text{ or } 113 \text{ mL/hr}$$

d. Titration factor
$$113 \text{ mL/hr} = 113 \text{ gtt/min}$$
$$\frac{300 \text{ mcg/min}}{113 \text{ gtt/min}} = 2.65 \text{ or } 3 \text{ mcg/gtt}$$

e.
$$7 \text{ gtt} \times 3 \text{ mcg/gtt} = 21 \text{ mcg}$$
$$21 \text{ mcg} + 300 \text{ mcg/min} = 321 \text{ mcg/min}$$
$$7 \text{ gtt} + 113 \text{ gtt/min} = 120 \text{ gtt/min or } 120 \text{ mL/hr}$$

f.
$$5 \text{ gtt} \times 3 \text{ mcg/gtt} = 15 \text{ mcg}$$
$$321 \text{ mcg/min} - 15 \text{ mcg} = 306 \text{ mcg/min}$$
$$120 \text{ gtt/min} - 5 \text{ gtt} = 115 \text{ gtt/min or } 115 \text{ mL/hr}$$

V. "Factor of 15" Method

1. $15 \times 74 \text{ kg} = 1110 \text{ mg}$

2. $15 \times 80 \text{ kg} = 1200 \text{ mg}$

VI. Total Amount of Drug Infused Over Time

1. Lidocaine bolus:
$$\begin{array}{r} 100 \text{ mg} \\ + \underline{100 \text{ mg}} \\ 200 \text{ mg} \end{array}$$

Lidocaine IV infusion:

a. Concentration of solution: given as 4 mg/mL in problem.

b. Concentration/hr:
$$4 \text{ mg/mL} \times 40 \text{ mL/hr} = 160 \text{ mg/hr}$$

c. Concentration over ½ hr:
$$160 \text{ mg/hr} \times \frac{30 \text{ min}}{60 \text{ min/hr}} = 80 \text{ mg over } 30 \text{ min}$$

d. Amount of IV drug infused:

Lidocaine per two boluses: 200 mg
Lidocaine per IV infusion: + $\underline{80 \text{ mg}}$
 280 mg total amount infused over 1 hr

Note: The infusion rate is close to exceeding the maximum therapeutic range, which is 200–300 mg/hr.

2. Concentration of solution

$$20,000 \text{ U} : 500 \text{ mL} :: X \text{ U} : 1 \text{ mL}$$
$$500 \text{ X} = 20,000$$
$$\text{X} = 40 \text{ U}$$

a. The concentration of solution is 40 U/mL.

b. Concentration/hr:

$$40 \text{ U/mL} \times 50 \text{ mL/hr} = 2000 \text{ U/hr}$$

c. Amount of IV drug infused over 5½ hours:

$$2000 \text{ U} \times \frac{30 \text{ min}}{60 \text{ min/hr}} = 1000 \text{ U over ½ hr}$$

$$200 \text{ U} \times 5 \text{ hr} = 10,000 \text{ U/5 hr}$$

$$\begin{array}{r} 10,000 \text{ U} \\ + \underline{1,000 \text{ U}} \\ 11,000 \text{ U over 5½ hr} \end{array}$$

Pediatric Critical Care

OBJECTIVES

- Recognize factors that contribute to errors in drug and fluid administration.
- Identify the steps in calculating dilution parameters.
- Determine the accuracy of the dilution parameters in a drug order.

In delivering emergency drugs with complex dilution calculations, it is important for the nurse to evaluate the accuracy of the physician's order and ensure that the child does not receive excessive fluids. Many institutions are attempting to standardize the concentration of the solution for various pediatric intravenous dosages to decrease the occurrence of miscalculations.

As noted in Chapter 10, the concepts of concentration of the solution, infusion rates for concentration and volume, and concentration of a drug for specific body weight per unit time are also used to prepare the pediatric dose.

FACTORS INFLUENCING INTRAVENOUS ADMINISTRATION

Excessive fluid can be given when the fluid volume of the emergency drug is not considered in the 24-hour fluid intake. Long intravenous (IV) tubing can be another source of fluid excess and can cause errors in drug delivery. When the priming or filling volume of the IV tubing is not considered, the child may receive extra fluid, especially if medication is added to the primary IV set via a secondary IV set. IV medication may not reach the child if the IV infusion rate is low, such as 1 mL/hr, or if the IV tubing has not been primed or filled with the medication prior to infusion. Most pediatric departments are developing protocols for safe and consistent IV drug delivery.

CALCULATING ACCURACY OF DILUTION PARAMETERS

The nurse may find it necessary to calculate the dilution parameters of a drug order that specifies the concentration/kg/min and the volume/hr infusion rate. The physician should determine all drug dose parameters, which include concentration/kg/min, volume/hr, and dilution parameters. The nurse should check the accuracy of the dilution parameters to ensure that the correct drug dosage is given. These methods are also used to prepare the pediatric dose. In many pediatric critical care areas, intravenous fluids for drug administration are limited to prevent fluid overload. If the physician changes the drug dosage, rather than increasing the volume (mL), the concentration of the solution may be changed.

EXAMPLES

PROBLEM 1: A 6-day-old infant, weight 3.5 kg, is in septic shock.
Order: dopamine 5 mcg/kg/min at 1 mL/hr and dilute as follows, 100 mg in 100 mL D₅½ NSS.
Dosage: 2–5 mcg/kg/min.
Drug available: dopamine 40 mg/mL

The following steps are needed to determine if dilution orders will give the correct concentration of solution to deliver 5 mcg/kg/min at 1 mL/hr.

Step 1: Determine infusion rates for concentration per unit time.

    1. Find the concentration per minute.

$$\text{infant weight} \times \text{concentration/kg/min} =$$
$$3.5 \text{ kg} \quad \times \quad 5 \text{ mcg/kg/min} \quad = 17.5 \text{ mcg/min}$$

    2. Calculate the concentration per hour.

$$17.5 \text{ mcg/min} \times 60 \text{ min/hr} = 1050 \text{ mcg/hr}$$

Step 2: Determine concentration of solution.
    Divide the concentration per hr by volume per hr.

$$\frac{1050 \text{ mcg/hr}}{1 \text{ mL/hr}} = 1050 \text{ mcg/mL or 1 mg/mL}$$

Step 3: Determine the accuracy of the dilution order.
    Find how much dopamine must be added to 100 mL
    Set up a ratio and proportion.

$$1 \text{ mg} \quad : \quad 1 \text{ mL} \; : : \; X \; : \quad 100 \text{ mL}$$
$$X = 100 \text{ mg}$$

Dilution order is correct.

PREPARATION OF DRUG DOSAGE:

$$\frac{D}{H} \times V = \frac{100}{40} \times 1 = 2.5 \text{ mL} \quad \textbf{or}$$

$$H \quad : \quad V \; : : \quad D \quad : \quad V$$
$$40 \text{ mg} \; : \; 1 \text{ mL} \; : : \; 100 \text{ mg} \; : \; X \text{ mL}$$
$$40 X = 100$$
$$X = 2.5 \text{ mL}$$

Answer: Add 2.5 mL of dopamine 40 mg/mL to 100 mL $D_5\frac{1}{2}$ NSS.

PROBLEM 2: A 3-week-old infant, weight 1.6 kg, is in septic shock.
    Order: dobutamine 2.5 mcg/kg/min by a syringe pump
    with a 35-mL syringe at 1 mL/hr.
    Dilution: dobutamine 8.4 mg with $D_5\frac{1}{4}$ NSS to equal
    35 mL.
    Dosage: 2.5–40 mcg/kg/min.
    Drug available: dobutamine 250 mg/20 mL.
    Determine accuracy of dilution order to deliver 2.5 mcg/
    kg/min at 1 mL/hr.

Step 1: Find the infusion rates for concentration per unit time.

    1. Determine the concentration per minute.

$$\text{Infant weight} \times \text{concentration/kg/min} =$$
$$1.6 \text{ kg} \quad \times \quad 2.5 \text{ mcg/kg/min} \quad = 4 \text{ mcg/min}$$

    2. Determine the concentration per hour.

$$4 \text{ mcg/min} \times 60 \text{ min/hr} = 240 \text{ mcg/hr}$$

Step 2: Determine the concentration of solution.
    Divide the concentration per hr by volume per hr.

$$\frac{240 \text{ mcg/hr}}{1 \text{ mL/hr}} = 240 \text{ mcg/mL}$$

Step 3: Determine the accuracy of the dilution order.
Find how much dobutamine must be added to make 35 mL.

$$240 \text{ mcg} \quad : \quad 1 \text{ mL} \quad :: \quad X \text{ mcg} \quad : \quad 35 \text{ mL}$$
$$X = 8400 \text{ mcg or } 8.4 \text{ mg}$$

The dilution order is correct.

PREPARATION OF DRUG DOSAGE:

$$\frac{D}{H} \times V = \frac{8.4 \text{ mg}}{250 \text{ mg}} \times 20 \text{ mL} = 0.672 \text{ mL}$$

or

$$250 \text{ mg} \quad : \quad 20 \text{ mL} \quad :: \quad 8.4 \text{ mg} \quad : \quad X \text{ mL}$$
$$250 \, X = 168$$
$$X = 0.67 \text{ mL}$$

Answer: Add 0.67 mL of dobutamine 250 mg/20 mL to 34.33 mL D$_5$¼ NSS.

PROBLEM 3: For the same infant, the physician increases the dose of dobutamine. Again fluids must be limited, and another concentration must be prepared.
Order: 15 mcg/kg/min by a syringe pump. Dilute 40.5 mg in 35 mL D$_5$¼ NSS and administer 1 mL/hr. Determine the accuracy of dilution order to deliver 15 mcg/kg/min at 1 mL/hr.

Step 1: Determine the infusion rates for concentration per unit time.

1. Find the concentration per minute.

$$\text{infant weight} \times \text{concentration/kg/min} =$$
$$1.6 \text{ kg} \quad \times \quad 15 \text{ mcg/kg/min} \quad = 24 \text{ mcg/min}$$

2. Find the concentration per hour.

$$24 \text{ mcg/min} \times 60 \text{ min/hr} = 1440 \text{ mcg/hr}$$

Step 2: Calculate the concentration of solution.
Divide the concentration per hr by volume per hr.

$$\frac{1440 \text{ mcg/hr}}{1 \text{ mL/hr}} = 1440 \text{ mcg/mL}$$

Step 3: Determine the accuracy of the dilution order.

$$1440 \text{ mcg} \quad : \quad 1 \text{ mL} \quad :: \quad X \text{ mcg} \quad : \quad 35 \text{ mL}$$
$$X = 50,400 \text{ mcg}$$

$$50,400 \text{ mcg} = 50.4 \text{ mg} \quad \text{or} \quad 50 \text{ mg}$$

Answer: The dilution order is *incorrect;* 50 mg of dobutamine is needed to deliver 15 mcg/kg/min.

SUMMARY PRACTICE PROBLEMS

Determine if dilution orders will yield the correct concentration of solution.

1. A 2-year-old child with acute status asthmaticus.
Child weighs 10.5 kg,
Order: aminophylline 110 mg in 500 mL of D_5W at 40 mL/hr.
Pediatric dose: 0.85 mg/kg/hr.
Drug available: aminophylline 250 mg/10 mL.

2. A 9-year-old child with supraventricular tachycardia.
Child weighs 30 kg.
Order: lidocaine 20 mcg/kg/min.
Dilute: 300 mg in 250 mL of D_5W at 30 mL/hr.
Pediatric dose: 20–40 mcg/kg/min.
Drug available: lidocaine 1 g/25 mL.

3. A 1-year-old child with septic shock.
Child weighs 9 kg.
Order: dopamine 5 mcg/kg/min.
Dilute: 100 mg in 200 mL of $D_5\frac{1}{4}$ NSS at 6.75 mL/hr.
Pediatric dose: 2–5 mcg/kg/min.
Drug available: dopamine 400 mg/5 mL.

4. A 3-year-old child in shock.
Child weighs 16 kg.
Order: sodium nitroprusside 2 mcg/kg/min.
Dilute: 25.25 mg in 250 mL of D_5W at 19 mL/hr.
Pediatric dose: 200–500 mcg/kg/hr.
Drug available: sodium nitroprusside 50 mg/5 mL.

5. A 10-year-old child with diabetic ketoacidosis.
Child weighs 32 kg.
Order: regular Humulin insulin 50 U in 500 mL of normal saline at 32 mL/hr.
Pediatric dose: 0.1 U/kg/hr.
Drug available: 100 U/mL.

ANSWERS

1. *Step 1:* Infusion rates for concentration.
Concentration per hour.

$$10.5 \text{ kg} \times 0.85 \text{ mg/kg/hr} = 8.9 \text{ mg/hr}$$

Step 2: Concentration of solution.

$$\frac{8.9 \text{ mg/hr}}{40 \text{ mL/hr}} = 0.22 \text{ mg/mL}$$

Step 3: Accuracy of dilution order.

$$\begin{array}{ccccccc} mg & : & mL & : : & mg & : & mL \\ 0.22 & : & 1 & : : & X & : & 500 \end{array}$$
$$X = 110 \text{ mg}$$

Dilution order is correct.

Preparation of drug dosage:

$$\frac{D}{H} \times V = \frac{110}{250} \times 10 = \frac{1100}{250} = 4.4 \text{ mL}$$

or

$$\begin{array}{ccccc} 250 \text{ mg} & : & 10 \text{ mL} & : : & 110 \text{ mg} \quad X \text{ mL} \end{array}$$
$$250 \text{ X} = 1100$$
$$X = 4.4 \text{ mL}$$

2. *Step 1:* Infusion rates for concentration/unit time.
  a. Concentration per minute.

$$30 \text{ kg} \times 20 \text{ mcg/kg/min} = 600 \text{ mcg/min}$$

  b. Concentration per hour.

$$600 \text{ mcg/min} \times 60 \text{ min/hr} = 36,000 \text{ mcg/hr}$$

Step 2: Concentration of solution.

$$\frac{36,000 \text{ mcg/hr}}{30 \text{ mL/hr}} = 1200 \text{ mcg/mL} \quad \text{or} \quad 1.2 \text{ mg/mL}$$

Step 3: Accuracy of dilution order.

$$\begin{array}{ccccccc} 1.2 \text{ mg} & : & 1 \text{ mL} & : : & X \text{ mg} & : & 250 \text{ mL} \end{array}$$
$$X = 300 \text{ mg}$$

Dilution order is correct.

Preparation of drug dosage:

$$\frac{D}{H} \times V = \frac{300}{1000} \times 25 = \frac{7500}{1000} = 7.5 \text{ mL}$$

or

$$\begin{array}{ccccccc} 1000 \text{ mg} & : & 25 \text{ mL} & : : & 300 \text{ mg} & : & X \text{ mL} \end{array}$$
$$1000 \text{ X} = 7500$$
$$X = 7.5 \text{ mL}$$

Answer: 7.5 mL of lidocaine added to 250 mL.

3. *Step 1:* Infusion rate for concentration.
  a. Concentration per minute.

$$9 \text{ kg} \times 5 \text{ mcg/kg/min} = 45 \text{ mcg/min}$$

  b. Concentration per hour.

$$45 \text{ mcg/min} \times 60 \text{ min/hr} = 2700 \text{ mcg/hr}$$

Step 2: Concentration of solution.

$$\frac{2700 \text{ mcg/hr}}{6.75 \text{ mL/hr}} = 400 \text{ mcg/mL}$$

Step 3: Accuracy of dilution order.

$$400 \text{ mcg} \quad : \quad 1 \text{ mL} \quad : : \quad X \text{ mcg} \quad : \quad 200 \text{ mL}$$
$$X = 80,000 \text{ mcg or } 80 \text{ mg in } 200 \text{ mL}$$

Dilution order is incorrect.

4. *Step 1:* Infusion rates for concentration.
   a. Concentration per minute.

$$16 \text{ kg} \times 2 \text{ mcg/kg/min} = 32 \text{ mcg/min}$$

   b. Concentration per hour.

$$32 \text{ mcg/min} \times 60 \text{ min/hr} = 1920 \text{ mcg/hr}$$

Step 2: Concentration of solution.

$$\frac{1920 \text{ mcg/hr}}{19 \text{ mL/hr}} = 101 \text{ mcg/mL}$$

Step 3: Accuracy of order.

$$101 \text{ mcg} \quad : \quad 1 \text{ mL} \quad : : \quad X \text{ mcg} \quad : \quad 250 \text{ mL}$$
$$X = 25,250 \text{ mcg or } 25.25 \text{ mg}$$

Dilution order is correct.

Preparation of drug dosage:

$$\frac{D}{H} \times V = \frac{25.25}{50} \times 5 = 2.52 \text{ mL}$$

or

$$50 \text{ mg} \quad : \quad 5 \text{ mL} \quad : : \quad 25.25 \text{ mg} \quad : \quad X \text{ mL}$$
$$50 \text{ X} = 126.25$$
$$X = 2.52 \text{ mL}$$

Answer: *2.52 mL of sodium nitroprusside added to 250 mL.*

5. *Step 1:* Infusion rate for concentration.
   Concentration per hour.

$$32 \text{ kg} \times 0.1 \text{ U/kg/hr} = 3.2 \text{ U/hr}$$

Step 2: Concentration of solution.

$$\frac{3.2 \text{ U/hr}}{32 \text{ mL/hr}} = 0.01 \text{ U/mL}$$

Step 3: Accuracy of dilution order.

$$0.1 \text{ U} \quad : \quad 1 \text{ mL} = X \text{ U} \quad : \quad 500 \text{ mL}$$
$$X = 50 \text{ U}$$

Dilution order is correct.

Preparation of drug dose:

$$\frac{D}{H} \times V = \frac{50 \text{ U}}{100 \text{ U}} \times 1 = 0.5 \text{ mL}$$

Answer: *50 U/0.5 mL—use a U-100 insulin syringe.*

CHAPTER 12

Labor and Delivery

OBJECTIVES

- State the complication related to IV fluid administration in the high-risk mother.
- Recognize the different types of fluid administration used in high-risk labors.
- Determine the infusion rates of a drug in solution when the drug is prescribed by concentration or volume.

Drug calculations for labor and delivery are the same as those used in critical care. Determining the concentration of the solution, infusion rates, and titration factors are the primary calculation skills used. Accurate calculations are essential, as is the monitoring of intravenous (IV) fluid intake for medications and anesthetic procedures. Impaired renal filtration in preeclampsia and the antidiuretic effect of tocolytic drugs make the monitoring of fluid intake vital. Accurate measurement of IV fluid intake along with pulmonary assessment can decrease the risk of fluid overload and the sequelae of acute pulmonary edema in the high-risk mother.

Physicians' orders and hospital protocols give specific guidelines for administering IV drugs. The nurse is responsible for managing the IV drug therapy, monitoring the patient's fluid balance, and assessing the patient's response to drug therapy.

FACTORS INFLUENCING INTRAVENOUS FLUID AND DRUG MANAGEMENT

The most important concept in labor and delivery is that the drugs given to the mother also affect the unborn baby. Therefore, the response of the patient and the unborn baby must be closely monitored. Vital signs, urine output, reflexes, and contraction patterns are the main indicators of the mother's status. For the fetus, fetal heart rate is the primary guide.

TITRATION OF MEDICATIONS WITH MAINTENANCE INTRAVENOUS FLUIDS

Women in labor receive IV fluids to prevent dehydration when oral intake is contraindicated. IV drugs are given to stimulate labor, treat preeclampsia, or inhibit preterm labor. Normally, the IV fluids that the patient receives are given at 100 to 125 mL/hr. A bolus of IV fluids, 200 to 500 mL, may be given to initially hydrate the mother, especially in preterm labor or prior to conductive anesthesia. Any IV medications that are given by titration are a part of the hourly IV rate. The patient will have a primary IV line and a secondary IV line for medications. All IV medications should be delivered by a volumetric pump, which ensures that the specified volume and correct dosage are delivered.

Titration of drugs is frequently done for high-risk mothers with preeclampsia and mothers experiencing preterm labor. The most common use of titration is in the induction or stimulation of labor. In the following example, an oxytocic drug is given, and the primary IV rate is adjusted with the secondary IV drug line to achieve a therapeutic effect and maintain adequate maternal hydration. Note that the drug is ordered to be given by concentration and that the infusion rates for volume per minute and hour must be determined.

Administration by Concentration

EXAMPLE

1. Give IV fluids at 100 mL/hr with $D_5\frac{1}{2}$ NSS.

2. Mix 10 U of oxytocin in 1000 NSS. Start at 5 mU/min, increase by 1 or

2 mU/min, q10min, until uterine contractions are 2 to 3 minutes apart. Do not exceed 40 mU/min.

Note: 1 Unit (U) = 1000 milliunits (mU)

Available: Secondary set:
               oxytocin 10 U/mL
               1000 mL NSS
               microdrip IV set 60 gtt/mL
               volumetric pump
        Primary set:
               1000 mL $D_5\frac{1}{2}$ NSS
               IV set drop factor 10 gtt/mL

For the *secondary* set IV, the following calculations must be made:

1. Concentration of solution.
2. Infusion rates: volume per minute and hour.
3. Titration factor in concentration per minute (mU/min).

For the *primary* IV, the following calculations must be made:

1. Drop rate per minute.
2. Balance primary IV flow with secondary IV rate to achieve 100 mL/hr.

SECONDARY IV (SEE CHAP. 6 FOR FORMULAS)

1. Concentration of solution:

$$10\ U\ :\ 1000\ mL\ :\ :\ X\ :\ 1\ mL$$
$$1000\ X = 10$$
$$X = 0.01\ U\ or\ 10\ mU$$

The concentration of solution is 10 mU/mL.

2. Infusion rates for volume:

$$\frac{concentration/minute}{concentration\ of\ solution} = volume/min \times 60\ minutes = volume/hr$$

Volume per minute   *Volume per hour*

$$\frac{1\ mU/min}{10\ mU/mL} = 0.1\ mL/min \times 60\ minutes = 6\ mL/hr$$

$$\frac{2\ mU/min}{10\ mU/mL} = 0.2\ mL/min \times 60\ minutes = 12\ mL/hr$$

$$\frac{5\ mU/min}{10\ mU/mL} = 0.5\ mL/min \times 60\ minutes = 30\ mL/hr$$

3. Titration factor (see Chap. 8): to increase the concentration by increments of 1 mU/min, the hourly rate on the volumetric pump must increase by 6 mL/hr. The titration factor for this problem is 6

mL/hr. To increase the concentration to a higher rate, multiply the rate of increase times 6 mL/hr. (Example: to increase infusion to 5 mU/min, multiply 5 by 6 mL = 30 mL/hr.)

For the secondary IV line, the concentration of the solution is 10 mU/mL of oxytocin, with the infusion rate of 30 mL/hr to be increased in increments of 6 to 12 mL every 10 minutes until contractions are 2 to 3 minutes apart.

PRIMARY IV

The secondary IV rate will start at 30 mL/hr; therefore, the primary rate will be 70 mL/hr. (A balance is needed to achieve 100 mL/hr.)

Drop rate using a 10 gtt/mL set is

$$\frac{70 \text{ mL/hr} \times 10 \text{ gtt/mL}}{60 \text{ minutes}} = 11.6 \text{ or } 12 \text{ gtt/min}$$

For every increase in rate from the secondary line, a corresponding decrease must be made with the primary IV line. If the rate of the secondary line exceeds the ordered hourly rate, the primary IV may be shut off completely. The concentration of the solution may be changed by the physician if the mother is receiving too much fluid.

Administration by Volume

In the previous example, the oxytocin was ordered to infuse by concentration (mU/min), which is the recommended method for patient safety. Sometimes in clinical practice, the infusion rate may be ordered by volume (mL/hr).

EXAMPLE

Mix 10 U of oxytocin in 1000 mL NSS. Start at 30 mL/hr, increase by 6 to 12 mL q10min until uterine contractions are 2 to 3 minutes apart. Do not exceed 40 mU/min.

To determine the concentration per hour of infusion, multiply concentration of the solution by volume/hr = concentration/hr:

$$10 \text{ mU/mL} \times 30 \text{ mL/hr} = 300 \text{ mU/hr}$$

To determine the concentration of the infusion per minute, divide:

$$\frac{\text{concentration/hr}}{60 \text{ min/hr}} = \text{concentration/min}$$

$$\frac{300 \text{ mU/hr}}{60 \text{ min/hr}} = 5 \text{ mU/min}$$

Therefore, oxytocin solution with a concentration of 10 mU/mL at 30 mL/hr will administer 5 mU/min of the drug.

INTRAVENOUS LOADING DOSE

Some situations require intravenous medications to be infused over a short period of time to obtain a serum level for a therapeutic effect. This type of IV drug administration is called a loading dose.

In the following example, a preeclampsia patient receives a loading dose of magnesium sulfate, followed by a maintenance dose of magnesium sulfate, via the secondary IV line. A primary IV line is also maintained after the loading dose is given. At the end of this example, the total IV intake is determined for an 8-hour period.

EXAMPLE

1. Mix magnesium sulfate 20 g in 1000 mL of D_5W.
2. Infuse 4 g over 20 minutes, then maintain at 1 g/hr.
3. Start D_5 LRS at 75 mL/hr after magnesium sulfate loading dose.

Available: Secondary set:
magnesium sulfate 50% (5 g in 10-mL ampules)
1000 mL D_5W
microdrip IV set 60 gtt/mL
volumetric pump
Primary set:
1000 mL D_5 LRS
IV set drop factor 10 gtt/mL

For the *secondary* IV, the following calculations must be made:

1. Dose of magnesium sulfate in IV.
2. Concentration of solution.
3. Volume of loading dose and flow rate for volumetric pump (see Chap. 8).
4. Infusion rate: volume per hour of magnesium sulfate infusion.

For the *primary* IV, the following calculation must be made:

1. Drop rate per minute.

For the total IV intake, the following solutions must be added:

1. Volume of loading dose.
2. Volume of secondary IV for 8 hours.
3. Volume of primary IV for 8 hours.

SECONDARY IV

1. $\dfrac{D}{H} \times V = \dfrac{20\ g}{5\ g} \times 10\ mL = 40\ mL$ of magnesium sulfate or 4 ampules

2. Concentration of solution:

$$20\ g = 20{,}000\ mg$$
$$20{,}000\ mg\quad :\quad 1000\ mL\quad ::\quad X\quad :\quad 1\ mL$$
$$1000\ X = 20{,}000$$
$$X = 20\ mg$$

The concentration of solution is 20 mg/mL.

3. Volume of loading dose:

$$4 \text{ g} = 4000 \text{ mg}$$
$$20 \text{ mg} \quad : \quad 1 \text{ mL} \quad :: \quad 4000 \text{ mg} \quad : \quad X \text{ mL}$$
$$20 \text{ X} = 4000$$
$$X = 200 \text{ mL}$$

Flow rate for volumetric pump:

$$200 \text{ mL} \div \frac{20 \text{ min}}{60 \text{ min/hr}} = 200 \times \frac{\overset{3}{\cancel{60}}}{\underset{1}{\cancel{20}}} = 600 \text{ mL/hr}$$

The rate on the volumetric pump for the 4 g infusion of magnesium sulfate over 20 minutes will be 600 mL/hr. If the pump cannot be adjusted to that rate, then the infusion rate must be monitored closely and the patient observed for response to drug therapy.

4. Infusion rate: volume per hour

$$1 \text{ g} = 1000 \text{ mg}$$

$$\frac{\text{concentration/hr}}{\text{concentration of solution}} = \text{volume/hr} \qquad \frac{100 \text{ mg/hr}}{20 \text{ mg/mL}} = 50 \text{ mL/hr}$$

The rate on the volumetric pump for the 1 g/hr infusion will be 50 mL/hr.

PRIMARY IV

After the loading dose of magnesium sulfate, the primary IV will run at 75 mL/hr.

Drop rate using a 10 gtt/mL set is

$$\frac{75 \text{ mL/hr} \times 10 \text{ gtt/min}}{60 \text{ min}} = 12.5 \text{ or } 13 \text{ gtt/min}$$

TOTAL IV INTAKE OVER 8 HOURS

Volume of loading dose		200 mL
Volume of secondary IV	50 mL × 8 =	400 mL
Volume of primary IV	75 mL × 8 =	+ 600 mL
		1200 mL

Because fluid overload is a potential problem for preeclampsia patients, all IV fluids must be calculated accurately.

INTRAVENOUS FLUID BOLUS

An IV fluid is a large volume of 200 to 500 mL of IV fluid infused over a short period of time (1 hour or less). A bolus may be given prior to conductive anesthesia or to a preterm patient in labor.

In the next example, calculate the flow rate of an IV bolus from the primary IV followed by an infusion of a tocolytic drug given by titration. At the end of this example, calculate the patient's fluid intake for 8 hours.

EXAMPLE

1. Start 1000 D$_5$ LRS at 300 mL/10 min, then reduce to 125 mL/hr.

2. Mix terbutaline 5 mg in 1000 mL of NSS; start at 10 mcg/min; increase 5 mcg/min q10min until contractions subside.

Available: Primary set:
  1000 mL D$_5$ LRS
  IV set drop factor 10 gtt/mL
 Secondary set:
  terbutaline 1 mg/mL
  500 mL NSS
  microdrip IV set 60 gtt/mL
  volumetric pump

For the *secondary* IV, the following calculations must be made:

1. The dose of terbutaline in IV.

2. Concentration of solution.

3. Infusion rates: volume per minute and hour.

4. Titration factor for 5 mcg/mL.

For the *primary* IV, determine the following:

1. Drop rate per minute for 300 mL over 10 minutes and 125 mL/hr.

2. Balance the primary IV with the secondary IV to achieve a rate of 125 mL/hr.

Total the IV fluids for 8 hours.

SECONDARY IV

1. $\dfrac{D}{H} \times V = \dfrac{5\ mg}{1\ mg} \times 1\ mL = 5\ mL$ of terbutaline or 5 ampules

2. Concentration of solution

$$5\ mg = 5000\ mcg$$
$$5000\ mcg\quad :\quad 1000\ mL\quad :\ :\ X\ mcg\quad :\quad 1\ mL$$
$$1000\ X = 5000$$
$$X = 5\ mcg$$

The concentration of solution is 5 mcg/mL.

3. Infusion rates: volume per minute and hour

$$\frac{10\ \cancel{mcg}/min}{5\ \cancel{mcg}/mL} = 2\ mL/min \times 60\ min/hr = 120\ mL/hr$$

4. Titration factor: to increase the concentration by increments of 5 mcg/min, the volume of the increment of change must be calculated per minute and hour:

$$\frac{\text{concentration/minute}}{\text{concentration of solution}} = \text{mL/min} \qquad \frac{5 \text{ mcg/min}}{5 \text{ mcg/mL}} = 1 \text{ mL/min}$$

$$\text{volume/min} \times 60 \text{ min/hr} = \text{volume/hr}$$
$$1 \text{ mL/min} \times 60 \text{ min/hr} = 60 \text{ mL/hr}$$

The titration factor is 1 mL/min or 60 mL/hr. Increasing or decreasing the infusion rate by 5 mcg/min will correspond to an increase or decrease in volume by 1 mL/min or 60 mL/hr.

PRIMARY IV

1. Drop rate for 300 mL over 10 minutes:

$$\frac{300 \text{ mL} \times \overset{1}{\cancel{10}} \text{ gtt/mL}}{\underset{1}{\cancel{10} \text{ min}}} = 300 \text{ gtt/min}$$

Since this rate is too fast to count, the flow must be monitored closely. Drop rate for 125 mL/hr:

$$\frac{125 \text{ ml} \times \overset{1}{\cancel{10}} \text{ gtt/mL}}{\underset{6}{\cancel{60} \text{ min}}} = 20.8 \text{ or } 21 \text{ gtt/min}$$

TOTAL IV INTAKE OVER 8 HOURS

Volume of loading dose		300 mL
Volume of primary set	125 mL × 8 =	1000 mL
Volume of secondary set	180 mL × 8 =	+ 1440 mL
		2740 mL

Assume an average of 180 mL/hr was given.

SUMMARY PRACTICE PROBLEMS

1. Preterm labor.
 a. Give NSS 500 mL over 15 minutes, then infuse at 100 mL/hr.
 b. If contractions are still regular, mix ritodrine 150 mg in 500 mL NSS. Infuse at 50 mcg/min and increase by 50 mcg q10min until contractions cease. Do not infuse more than 350 mcg/min.

 Available: Primary set:
 1000 mL NSS
 IV set with drop factor of 10 gtt/mL
 Secondary set:
 ritodrine 50 mg in 5-mL ampules
 500 mL NSS
 microdrip set 60 gtt/mL
 volumetric pump

Determine the following:

a. Secondary IV:
  (1) Ritodrine dosage.
  (2) Concentration of solution.
  (3) Infusion rate for volume per minute and hour.
  (4) Titration factor.
b. Primary IV: drop rate for 500 mL over 15 minutes and 100 mL/hr.
c. Total fluid intake for 8 hours.

2. Preeclamptic labor.
  a. Mix magnesium sulfate 20 g in 1000 mL D_5W.
  b. Infuse 4 g over 30 minutes, then maintain at 2 g/hr.
  c. Start LRS 1000 mL at 50 mL/hr after loading dose of magnesium sulfate.

Available: Secondary set:
            magnesium sulfate 50% (5 g in 10 mL)
            1000 mL D_5W
            microdrip IV set 60 gtt/mL
            volumetric pump
        Primary set:
            1000 mL LRS
            IV set 10 gtt/mL

Determine the following:

a. Secondary IV:
  (1) Magnesium sulfate dosage.
  (2) Concentration of solution.
  (3) Volume of loading dose and infusion rate for volumetric pump.
  (4) Infusion rate per hour of magnesium sulfate.
b. Primary IV: drop rate for 50 mL/hr.
c. Total fluid intake for 8 hours.

ANSWERS

1. a. Secondary IV:
  (1) Ritodrine dosage:

$$\frac{D}{H} \times V = \frac{150 \text{ mg}}{50 \text{ mg}} \times 5 \text{ mL} = 15 \text{ mL}$$

   Add 15 mL or 3 ampules of ritodrine to 500 mL NSS.
  (2) Concentration of solution:

$$150 \text{ mg} \quad : \quad 500 \text{ mL} \quad : : \quad X \text{ mg} \quad : \quad 1 \text{ mL}$$
$$500 \text{ X} = 150$$
$$\text{X} = 0.3 \text{ mg/mL}$$

or

300 mcg/mL

(3) Infusion rates: volume per minute and hour

$$\frac{50 \text{ mcg/min}}{300 \text{ mcg/mL}} = 0.16 \text{ mL/min} \times 60 \text{ min/hr} = 9.6 \text{ or } 10 \text{ mL/hr}$$

(4) Titration factor: because the increment of increase is 50 mcg/min, the volume per hour, 10 mL/hr, is the titration factor, which increases the concentration by 50 mcg.

b. Primary IV:
(1) Drop rate for 500 mL over 15 minutes:

$$\frac{500 \text{ mL} \times 10 \text{ gtt/mL}}{15 \text{ min}} = 333 \text{ gtt/min}$$

This rate is impossible to count. Therefore, the infusion must be monitored closely during infusion time.

Drop rate for 100 mL/hr:

$$\frac{100 \text{ mL} \times 10 \text{ gtt/mL}}{60 \text{ min}} = 16.6 \text{ or } 17 \text{ gtt mL}$$

c. Total IV intake for 8 hours:

IV fluid bolus	500 mL
Primary IV 100 mL × 8 hr	800 mL
Secondary IV 50 mL × 8 hr	+ 400 mL
	1700 mL

Assume an average of 50 mL/hr was given.

2. a. Secondary IV:
(1) Magnesium sulfate dosage:

$$\frac{D}{H} \times V = \frac{20 \text{ mg}}{5 \text{ g}} \times 10 \text{ mL} = 40 \text{ mL or 4 ampules of magnesium sulfate}$$

(2) Concentration of solution:

$$20 \text{ g} = 200,000 \text{ mg}$$
$$20,000 \text{ mg} \quad : \quad 1000 \text{ mL} \quad : : \quad X \text{ mg} \quad : \quad 1 \text{ mL}$$
$$1000 X = 20,000$$
$$X = 20 \text{ mg}$$

The concentration of solution is 20 mg/mL.

(3) Volume of loading dose:

$$4 \text{ g} = 4000 \text{ mg}$$
$$20 \text{ mg} \quad : \quad 1 \text{ mL} \quad : : \quad 4000 \text{ mg} \quad : \quad X \text{ mL}$$
$$20 X = 4000$$
$$X = 200 \text{ mL}$$

Infusion rate for 30 minutes:

$$200 \text{ mL} \div \frac{30 \text{ min}}{60 \text{ min/hr}} = 200 \times \frac{\overset{2}{\cancel{60}}}{\underset{1}{\cancel{30}}} = 400 \text{ mL/hr}$$

CHAPTER 12 🖊 *Labor and Delivery* **261**

(4) Infusion rate: volume per hour

$$2\text{ g} = 2000\text{ mg}$$

$$\frac{2000\text{ mg/hr}}{20\text{ mg/mL}} = \text{mL/hr}$$

b. Primary IV:
After the loading dose

$$\frac{50\text{ mL/hr} \times 10\text{ gtt/min}}{60\text{ min}} = 8.3\text{ or } 8\text{ gtt/min}$$

c. Total IV intake over 8 hours:

Volume of loading dose		200 mL
Volume of secondary IV	100 mL × 8 =	800 mL
Volume of primary IV	50 mL × 8 =	+ 400 mL
		1400 mL

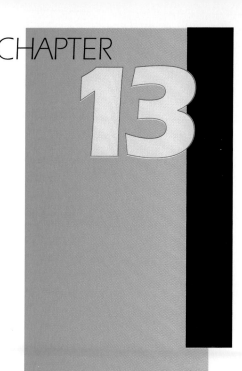

Community

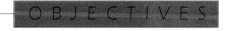

OBJECTIVES

- Identify the problems with conversion of metric to household measure.
- Name the components of a solution.
- List three methods for preparing a solution.
- Recognize three ways solutions are labeled.
- State the formula used for calculating a solution of a desired concentration.
- State the formula used for calculating a weaker solution from a stronger solution.

Although the metric system has become widespread in the clinical area, the home setting generally does not have the devices of metric measure. This becomes a problem when liquid medication is prescribed in metric measure for the home patient. The community nurse should be able to assist the client in converting metric to household measure when necessary.

Preparation of solutions in the home setting may involve conversion between the metric and household systems. Solutions used in the home setting can be used for oral fluid replacement, topical application, irrigation, or disinfection. Although the majority of the solutions are commercially available, solutions that can be prepared in the home can be effective and less costly than the premixed items.

When commercially prepared drugs are too concentrated for the client's use and must be diluted, it becomes necessary to calculate the strength of the solution to meet the therapeutic need as prescribed by the physician. Knowledge of solution preparation and metric–household conversion can be a useful skill for the community nurse.

METRIC TO HOUSEHOLD CONVERSION

When changing from metric to household measure, the ounce from the apothecary system is used as an intermediary, because there is no clear conversion between the two systems.

The conversion factors for volume are:

Ounces to milliliters: multiply ounces times 29.57

Milliliters to ounces: multiply milliliters times 0.034

The conversion factors for weight are:

Ounces to grams: multiply ounces times 28.35

Grams to ounces: multiply grams times 0.035

TABLE 13–1
Household to Metric Conversions

STANDARD HOUSEHOLD MEASURE	APOTHECARY	METRIC VOLUME	METRIC WEIGHT
⅛ teaspoon	7–8 gtt/¹⁄₄₈ oz	0.6 mL	0.6 g
¼ teaspoon	15 gtt/¹⁄₂₄ oz	1.25 mL	1.25 g
½ teaspoon	30 gtt/¹⁄₁₂ oz	2.5 mL	2.5 g
1 teaspoon	60 gtt/⅙ oz	5 mL	5 g
1 tablespoon/3 teaspoons	½ oz	15 mL	15 g
2 tablespoons/6 teaspoons	1 oz	¼ dL/30 mL	30 g
¼ cup/4 tablespoons	2 oz	½ dL/60 mL	55 g
⅓ cup/5 tablespoons	2½ oz	¾ dL/75 mL	75 g
½ cup	4 oz	1 dL/120 mL	110 g
1 cup	8 oz	¼ L/240–250 mL	225 g
1 pint	16 oz	½ L/480–500 mL	
1 quart	32 oz	1 L/1000 mL	
2 quarts/½ gallon	64 oz	2 L/2000 mL	
1 gallon	128 oz	3¾ L/3840–4000 mL	

   Note that weight and volume measures differ in the metric system. The properties of crystals, powders, and other solids account for the differences more so than do liquids. Also, as liquid measures increase in volume, there are greater discrepancies between metric and standard household measure. Table 13–1 shows the current approximate equivalents. Deciliters and liters are also included with the volume measurements. These terms will be seen more frequently as the use of the metric system increases. Although conversion charts are helpful guides, a metric measuring device would be optimal for drug administration. Standard household measuring devices should be used instead of tableware if a metric device is not available.

Practice Problems

Use Table 13–1 to convert metric to household measure.

   1. Dimetapp 2.5 mL every 6 hours as necessary.

   _____

   2. Ceclor 5 mL fours times per day.

   _____

   3. Tylenol elixir 1.25 mL every 6 hours as necessary for temperature greater than 102°F.

   _____

   4. Maalox 30 mL after meals and at bedtime.

   _____

   5. Neo-Calglucon 7.5 mL three times per day.

   _____

   6. Basaljel 45 mL after each meal.

   _____

   7. Castor oil 60 mL at bedtime.

   _____

   8. Metamucil 5 g in 1 glass of water every morning.

   _____

   9. Dilantin-30 suspension 10 mL twice per day.

   _____

   10. Homemade pediatric electrolyte solution:

   H_2O 1 L, boiled _____

   Sugar 30 g _____

   Salt 1.5 g _____

   Lite salt 2.5 g _____

   Baking soda 2.5 g _____

ANSWERS

1. Dimetapp 2.5 mL = ½ t
2. Ceclor 5 mL = 1 t
3. Tylenol elixir 1.25 mL = ¼ t
4. Maalox 30 mL = 2 T
5. Neo-Calglucon 7.5 mL = 1½ t
6. Basaljel 45 mL = 3 T
7. Castor oil 60 mL = 4 T or ¼ c
8. Metamucil 5 g = 1 t
9. Dilantin-30 suspension 10 mL = 2 t
10. H_2O 1 L = 1 qt
    Sugar 30 g = 2 T
    Salt 1.25 g = ¼ t
    Lite salt 2.5 g = ½ t
    Baking soda 2.5 g = ½ t

PREPARING A SOLUTION OF A DESIRED CONCENTRATION

All solutions contain a solute (drug) and a solvent (liquid). Solutions can be mixed three different ways:

1. *Weight to Weight:* Involves mixing the weight of a given solute with the weight of a given liquid.

Example: 5 g sugar with 100 g H_2O

This type of preparation is used in the pharmaceutical setting and is the *most accurate*. Scales for weight to weight preparation are not usually found in the home setting.

2. *Weight to Volume:* Uses the weight of a given solute with the volume of an appropriate amount of solvent.

Example: 10 g of salt in 1 L of H_2O

or

2 oz of salt in 1 qt of H_2O

Again, a scale is needed for this preparation.

3. *Volume to Volume:* Means a given volume of solution is mixed with a given volume of solution.

Example: 10 mL of hydrogen peroxide 3% in 1 dL H_2O

or

2 T of hydrogen peroxide 3% in ½ c H_2O

Preparing solutions volume to volume is commonly used in both the clinical and home setting.

After a solution is prepared, the strength can be expressed numerically in three different ways:

1. A ratio—1 : 20 acetic acid

2. A fraction—5 g/100 mL acetic acid

3. A percentage—5% acetic acid

With a ratio, the first number is the solute and the second number is the solvent. In a fraction, the numerator is the drug and the denominator is the liquid. A solution labeled by percentage indicates the amount of solute in 100 mL of liquid. All pharmaceutically prepared solutions use the metric system, and the ratio, fraction, and percentages are interpreted in *grams per milliliter.*

Changing a Ratio to Fractions and Percentage

A ratio can be changed to a percentage or a fraction by setting up a proportion using the following variables:

known drug : known volume : : desired drug : desired volume

A proportion can also be set up like a fraction:

$$\frac{known\ drug}{known\ volume} = \frac{desired\ drug}{desired\ volume}$$

REMEMBER: Any variable in this formula can be found if the other three variables are known.

EXAMPLE

PROBLEM 1: Change acetic acid 1 : 20 to a percentage

$$1\ g : 20\ mL = X\ g : 100\ mL$$
$$20\ X = 100$$
$$X = 5\ g$$
$$1\ g : 20\ mL = 5\ g : 100\ mL$$

Note: In percentage, the volume of liquid is 100 mL.

The ratio can be expressed as a fraction, 5 g/100 mL, or as a percentage, 5%. Another method of changing a ratio to a percentage involves finding a multiple of 100 for volume (denominator), then multiplying both terms by that multiple.

Practice Problems

Change the following ratios to fractions and percentages.

1. 4 : 1

2. 2 : 1

3. 1 : 50

4. 1 : 3

5. 1 : 1000

6. 1 : 10,000

7. 1 : 4

8. 1 : 5000

9. 1 : 200

10. 1 : 10

ANSWERS

1. $4:1 = X:100$
$X = 400$

$\dfrac{400}{100}$, 400%

2. $2:1 = X:100$
$X = 200$

$\dfrac{200}{100}$, 200%

3. $1:50 = X:100$
$50\,X = 100$
$X = 2$

$\dfrac{2}{100}$, 2%

4. $1:3 = X:100$
$3\,X = 100$
$X = 33.3$

$\dfrac{33.3}{100}$, 33.3%

5. $1:1000 = X:100$
$1000\,X = 100$
$X = 0.1$

$\dfrac{0.1}{100}$, 0.1%

6. $1:10,000 = X:100$
$10,000\,X = 100$
$X = 0.01$

$\dfrac{1}{10,000}$, 0.01%

7. $1:4 = X:100$
$4\,X = 100$
$X = 25$

$\dfrac{25}{100}$, 25%

8. $1:5000 = X:100$
$5000\,X = 100$
$X = 0.02$

$\dfrac{0.02}{100}$, 0.02%

9. $1:200 = X:100$
$200\,X = 100$
$X = 0.5$

$\dfrac{0.5}{100}$, 0.5%

10. $1:10 = X:100$
$10\,X = 100$
$X = 10$

$\dfrac{10}{100}$, 10%

In the previous problems, grams per milliliter is the unit of measure used for preparing solutions. Scales for measuring grams are rarely found in the clinical area or the home environment. Volume (mL) is the common measurement of drugs for administration. Drugs that are powders, crystals, and liquids are measured in graduated measuring cups with metric, apothecary, or household units. The milliliter, although a volume measure, can be substituted for a gram, a measure of mass, because at 4°C, 1 mL of water weighs 1 g. Mass and volume differ with the type of substance; thus, grams and milliliters are not exact equivalents in all instances, but they can be accepted as approximate values for solution preparation.

Calculating a Solution from a Ratio

To obtain a solution from a ratio, use the proportion or fraction method.

EXAMPLES

PROBLEM 1: Prepare 500 mL of a 1 : 100 vinegar–water solution for a vaginal douche.

known drug : known volume : : desired drug : desired volume
1 mL   :   100 mL   : :   X mL   :   500 mL
$100\,X = 500$
$X = 5\ \text{mL}$

or

$$\frac{\text{known drug}}{\text{known volume}} = \frac{\text{desired drug}}{\text{desired volume}}$$

$$\frac{1\ \text{mL}}{100\ \text{mL}} = \frac{X}{500\ \text{mL}}$$

$$100\,X = 500$$
$$X = 5\ \text{mL}$$

Answer: 5 mL of vinegar added to 500 mL of water is a 1 : 100 vinegar–water solution.

Note: Five milliliters did not increase the volume of the solution by a large amount. When mixing volume and volume solutions, the total amount of *desired volume* should not be exceeded. Therefore, it is important to determine the volume of desired drug first, then remove that volume from the appropriate amount of solvent (solution). When mixing the solution, begin with the desired drug and add the premeasured solvent. This process will ensure that the solution has an accurate concentration.

PROBLEM 2: Prepare 100 mL of a 1 : 4 hydrogen peroxide 3% and normal saline mouthwash.

known drug : known volume : : desired drug : desired volume
1 mL   :   4 mL   : :   X mL   :   100 mL
$$4 X = 100 \text{ mL}$$
$$X = 25 \text{ mL}$$

25 mL of hydrogen peroxide 3% is the amount of desired drug. To calculate the amount of normal saline, use the following formula:

desired volume − desired drug = desired solvent
100 mL   −   25 mL   =   75 mL

Answer: 75 mL of saline and 25 mL of hydrogen peroxide 3% make 100 mL of a 1 : 4 mouthwash.

Calculating a Solution from a Percentage

To obtain a solution from a percentage, use the same formula with either the proportion or fraction method.

EXAMPLE

PROBLEM 1: Prepare 1000 mL of a 0.9% NaCl solution.

known drug : known volume : : desired drug : desired volume
0.9 g   :   100 mL   : :   X g   :   1000 mL
$$100 X = 900$$
$$X = 9 \text{ g or } 9 \text{ mL}$$

Answer: 9 g or 9 mL of NaCl in 1000 mL will make a 0.9% NaCl solution.

PREPARING A WEAKER SOLUTION FROM A STRONGER SOLUTION

When a situation requires the preparation of a weaker solution from a stronger solution, the amount of desired drug must be determined. The known variables are the desired solution, the available or on-hand solution, and the desired volume. The formula can be set up with the strength of the solutions expressed in either ratio or percentage. The proportion method or the fractional method can be used to solve the problem. The first ratio or fraction, the desired solution (weaker solution), is the numerator, and the available or on-hand solution (stronger solution) is the denominator.

desired solution : available solution : : desired drug : desired volume

or

$$\frac{\text{desired solution}}{\text{available solution}} = \frac{\text{desired drug}}{\text{desired volume}}$$

EXAMPLE

PROBLEM 1: Prepare 500 mL of a 2.5% aluminum acetate solution from a 5% aluminum acetate solution. Use water as the solvent.

2.5% : 5% : : X : 500 mL
2.5 mL : 5 mL : : X : 500 mL
5 X = 1250
X = 250 mL

Answer: Use 250 mL of 5% aluminum acetate to make 500 mL of 2.5% aluminum acetate solution.

Determine the amount of water needed.

desired volume − desired drug = desired solvent
500 mL   −   250 mL   =   250 mL

or

Same problem using the fractional method:

$$\frac{2.5\%}{5\%} \times \frac{X}{500 \text{ mL}} =$$

5 X = 1250
X = 250 mL of 5% aluminum acetate

or

Same problem but stated as a ratio:

Prepare 500 mL of a 1 : 40 aluminum acetate solution from a 1 : 20 aluminum acetate solution with water as the solvent.

$$\frac{1}{40} : \frac{1}{20} : : X : 500 \text{ mL}$$

$$\frac{1}{20\,X} = \frac{500}{40}$$

$$X = \frac{500}{\overset{40}{\underset{2}{}}} \times \frac{\overset{1}{2\!\!\!0}}{1} = \frac{500}{2}$$

X = 250 mL of 5% aluminum acetate solution

GUIDELINES FOR HOME SOLUTIONS

For solutions prepared by clients in the home, directions need to be very specific and in written form, if possible. People often think that more is better. Teach the client that solutions can be dangerous if they are too concentrated. Higher concentrations of solutions can irritate tissues and prevent the desired effect. Recommend that standard measuring spoons and cups be used rather than tableware. Level measures rather than heaping measures of dry solutes should be used. Utensils and containers for solution preparation should be *clean or sterilized by boiling* if used for infants. Avoid mixing acidic solutions in aluminum containers, especially if the solution is for oral use. Although there is no evidence of toxicity, a metallic taste is noticeable. Glass, enamel, or plastic containers can be used. Solutions should be made fresh daily or prior to use. Oral solutions, especially for infants, require refrigeration; this is not necessary for topical solutions.

When preparing the solution, start with the desired drug and then add the solvent. This helps to disperse the drug and ensures that the desired volume of solution is not exceeded.

Solution problems are best calculated within the metric system. Fractional and percentage dosages are difficult to determine within the household system.

Summary Practice Problems

Identify the known variables and choose the appropriate formula. Calculate the following solutions using the metric system. Use the conversion table to obtain the household equivalent.

1. Prepare 250 mL of a 0.6% NaCl and sterile water solution for nose drops.

   _____

2. Prepare 250 mL of a 5% glucose and sterile water solution for an infant feeding.

   _____

3. Prepare 100 mL of a 25% Betadine solution with sterile saline for a foot soak.

   _____

4. Prepare 2 L of a 2% Lysol solution for cleaning a changing area.

   _____

5. Prepare 20 L of a 2% sodium bicarbonate solution for a bath.

   _____

6. Prepare 100 mL of a 50% hydrogen peroxide 3% and water mouthwash.

   _____

7. Prepare 500 mL of a modified Dakin's solution 0.5% from a 5% sodium hypochlorite solution with sterile water as the solvent.

_____

8. Prepare 1500 mL of a 0.9% NaCl solution for an enema.

_____

9. Prepare 2 L of a 1 : 1000 Neosporin bladder irrigation with sterile saline. (Omit the household conversion.)

_____

10. Determine how much alcohol is needed for a 3 : 1 alcohol and white vinegar solution for an external ear irrigation. Vinegar 30 mL is used. Solve using the proportion method.

_____

11. Prepare 1000 mL of a 1 : 10 sodium hypochlorite and water solution for cleaning.

_____

12. Prepare 1000 mL of a 3% sodium hypochlorite and water solution.

_____

ANSWERS

1. Known drug: 0.6% NaCl   0.6 : 100 : : X : 250
   Known volume: 100 mL   100 X = 150
   Desired drug: X   X = 1.5 mL
   Desired volume: 250 mL

   1.5 mL of NaCl in 250 mL of water yields a 0.6% NaCl solution. Household equivalents are approximately ¼ teaspoon salt and 1 cup sterile water.

2. Known drug: 5% glucose (sugar)   5 : 100 : : X : 250
   Known volume: 100 mL   100 X = 1250
   Desired drug: X   X = 12.5 mL
   Desired volume: 250 mL

   12.5 mL of sugar in 250 mL of water yields a 5% glucose solution. Household equivalents are approximately 1 tablespoon in 1 cup of sterile water.

3. Known drug: 25% Betadine   25 : 100 : : X : 1000
   Known volume: 100 mL   100 X = 25,000
   Desired drug: X   X = 250 mL
   Desired volume: 1000 mL   100 mL − 250 mL = 250 mL

   250 mL of Betadine in 750 mL saline yields a 25% Betadine solution. Household equivalents are 1 cup Betadine in 3 cups sterile saline.

4. Known drug: 2% Lysol   2 : 100 : : X : 2000 mL
   Known volume: 100 mL   100 X = 4000
   Desired drug: X   X = 40 mL
   Desired volume: 2 L = 2000 mL

   40 mL of Lysol in 2 L of water yields a 2% Lysol solution. Household equivalents are 2 tablespoons and 2 teaspoons (40 mL) of Lysol to 2 quarts or ½ gallon of water.

5. Known drug: 2% sodium bicarbonate $2:100::X:20,000$ mL
    Known volume: 100 mL $X = 40,000$
    Desired drug: X $X = 400$ mL or 400 g
    Desired volume: 20,000 mL

400 mL or 400 g of sodium bicarbonate (baking soda) in 20,000 mL of water yields a 2% sodium bicarbonate solution. Household equivalents are 1½ cups and 2 tablespoons baking soda in 5 gallons of water.

6. Known drug: 50% hydrogen peroxide $50:100::X:100$
    Known volume: 100 mL $100\,X = 5000$
    Desired drug: X $X = 50$ mL
    Desired volume: 100 mL 100 mL $- 50$ mL $= 50$ mL

50 mL of hydrogen peroxide 3% in 50 mL water yields a 50% solution. Household equivalents are approximately 3 tablespoons of hydrogen peroxide 3% in 3 tablespoons of water.

7. Desired solution: 0.5% $0.5:5::X:500$
    Available solution: 5% $5\,X = 250$
    Desired drug: X $X = 50$ mL
    Desired volume: 500 mL 500 mL $- 50$ mL $= 450$ mL

50 mL of sodium hypochlorite in 450 mL sterile water yields a 0.5% modified Dakin's solution. Household equivalents are 3 tablespoons and 1 teaspoon of Dakin's solution in 1 pint minus 3 tablespoons of water.

8. Known drug: 0.9% $0.9:100::X:1500$
    Known volume: 100 mL $100\,X = 1350$
    Desired drug: X $X = 13.5$ mL
    Desired volume: 1500 mL

13.5 mL of NaCl in 1500 mL water yields a 0.9% NaCl solution. Household equivalents are 2½ teaspoons of salt in 1½ quarts of water.

9. Known drug: 1 mL $1:1000::X:2000$
    Known volume: 1000 mL $1000\,X = 2000$
    Desired drug: X $X = 2$ mL
    Desired volume: 2000 mL

2 mL of Neosporin irrigant in 2000 mL sterile saline yields a 1:1000 solution for continuous bladder irrigation. This treatment is done primarily in the clinical setting.

10. Use ratio and proportion to solve this problem.

$$3:1::X:30 \text{ mL}$$
$$X = 90 \text{ mL}$$

Add 90 mL of alcohol to 30 mL of vinegar to yield a 3:1 solution for an external ear wash. Household equivalents are 6 tablespoons of alcohol and 2 tablespoons of vinegar.

11. Known drug: 1 mL $1:10::X:1000$
    Known volume: 10 mL $10\,X = 1000$
    Desired drug: X $X = 100$ mL
    Desired volume: 1000 mL 1000 mL $- 100$ mL $= 900$ mL

100 mL of sodium hypochlorite (bleach) in 900 mL water yields a 1:10 sodium hypochlorite solution. Household equivalents are ⅓ cup and 2 tablespoons sodium hypochlorite in approximately 1 quart minus ⅓ cup and 2 tablespoons of water.

12. Known drug: 3 mL 3 : 100 : : X : 1000

Known volume: 100 mL 100 X = 3000

Desired drug: X X = 30 mL

Desired volume: 1000 mL 1000 mL − 30 mL = 970 mL

30 mL of sodium hypochlorite (bleach) in 970 mL water yields a 3% sodium hypochlorite solution. Household equivalents are 2 tablespoons in 1 quart minus 2 tablespoons of water.

Akers, M. J. (1987). Considerations in using the IV route for drug delivery. *American Journal of Hospital Pharmacy.* 44:2528–2530.

Axton, S. E., and Fugate, T. (1987). A protocol for pediatric IV meds. *American Journal of Nursing.* 7:943–945.

Barnhart, E. R. (1991). *Physician's Desk Reference (PDR).* 45th edition. Oradell, NJ: Medical Economics.

Behrman, R. E., and Vaughan, V. C. (1987). *Nelson Textbook of Pediatrics.* 13th edition. Philadelphia: W. B. Saunders.

Biller, J., and Yeager, A. (eds.) (1981). *The Harriet Land Handbook.* 9th edition. Chicago: Year Book Medical Publishers.

Carey, B. (1982). Microdrop calculations for neonates in converting micrograms/kilograms/minute to microdrops. *Dimensions of Critical Care Nursing.* 6:338–339.

Colangelo, A. (1987). Drug preparation techniques for IV drug delivery systems. *American Journal of Hospital Pharmacy.* 44(11):2550–2553.

Comer, J. (1981). *Pharmacology in Critical Care.* Bethany, CT: Fleschner Publishing.

Daniels, J. M., and Smith, L. M. (1990). *Clinical Calculations.* 2nd edition. Albany, NY: Delmar Publishers.

DeAngelis, R., and Brott, W. (1982). The "factor 15" method in converting micrograms/kilograms/minute to microdrops. *Dimensions of Critical Care Nursing.* 6:334–337.

Deglin, J. H. (1988). *Dosage Calculations Manual.* Springhouse, PA: Springhouse.

Deglin, J. H., Vallerand, A. H., and Russin, M. M. (1991). *Davis's Drug Guide for Nurses.* 2nd edition. Philadelphia: F. A. Davis.

Edmunds, M. W. (1991). *Introduction to Clinical Pharmacology.* St. Louis: C. V. Mosby.

Estoup, M. (1994). Approaches and limitations of medication delivery in patients with enteral feeding tubes. *Critical Care Nurse.* 14(1): 68–79.

Gilman, A. G., Goodman, L. S., and Gilman, A. (eds.) (1991). *Goodman and Gilman's The Pharmacological Basis of Therapeutics.* 8th edition. New York: Pergamon Press.

Howry, L. B., Bindler, R. M., and Tso, Y. (1981). *Pediatric Medications.* Philadelphia: J. B. Lippincott.

Huey, F. (1983). What's on the market? A nurse's guide. *American Journal of Nursing.* 6:902–910.

IV Therapy. Clinical Skillbuilders. (1990). Springhouse, PA: Springhouse.

Katzung, B. G. (1992). *Basic and Clinical Pharmacology.* 5th edition. Norwalk, CT: Appleton & Lange.

Kee, J. L., and Hayes, E. R. (1993). *Pharmacology: A Nursing Process Approach.* Philadelphia: W. B. Saunders.

Kee, J. L., and Paulanka, B. J. (1994). *Fluids and Electrolytes with Clinical Applications.* 5th edition. Albany, NY: Delmar Publishing.

Keenan, P. (1982). The "key number" conversion method in converting micrograms/kilograms/minute to microdrops. *Dimensions of Critical Care Nursing.* 6:332–333.

Leff, R. D. (1987). Features of IV devices and equipment that affect IV drug delivery. *American Journal of Hospital Pharmacy.* 44(11):2530–2533.

Lilley, L. L., and Guanci, R. (1994). Getting back to basics. *American Journal of Nursing.* 9:15, 16.

Medication Administration and IV Therapy Manual (1988). Springhouse, PA: Springhouse.

Miyagawa, C. I. (1993). Drug-nutrient interactions in critically ill patients. *Critical Care Nurse.* 13:69–87.

Loebl, S., Spratto, G., and Woods, A. (1989). *The Nurse's Drug Handbook.* 5th edition. New York: John Wiley and Sons.

Norton, B. A., and Miller, A. M. (1986). *Skills for Professional Nursing Practice.* Norwalk, CT: Appleton-Century-Crofts.

Piecoro, J. J. (1987). Development of an institutional IV drug delivery policy. *American Journal of Hospital Pharmacy.* 44(11):2557–2559.

Rapp, R. P. (1987). Considering product features and costs in selecting a system for intermittent IV drug delivery. *American Journal of Hospital Pharmacy.* 44(11):2533–2538.

Reilly, K. M. (1987). Problems in administration techniques and dose measurement that influence accuracy of IV drug delivery. *American Journal of Hospital Pharmacy.* 44(11):2545–2550.

Rimar, J. M. (1987). Guidelines for the intravenous administration of medications used in pediatrics. *Maternal Child Nursing.* 12(5):322–340.

Rosenthal, K. (1982). Charts vs formula method in converting micrograms/kilograms/minute to microdrops. *Dimensions of Critical Care Nursing.* 6:326–331.

Roth-Skidmore, L. (1993). *Mosby's 1993 Nursing Drug Reference.* St. Louis: C. V. Mosby.

Russell, H. (1980). *Pediatric Drugs and Nursing Interventions.* New York: McGraw-Hill.

Smith, A. J. (1989). *Dosage and Solutions Calculations.* St. Louis: C. V. Mosby.

Spratto, G. R., and Woods, A. L. (1995). *Nurse's Drug Reference (NDR 95).* Albany, NY: Delmar Publishers.

Vallerand, A. H., and Deglin, J. H. (1991). *Nurse's Guide for IV Medications.* Philadelphia: F. A. Davis.

Weyant, H. (1984). Utilization of an intravenous drug guide. *Focus on Critical Care.* 2:58–62.

Wilson, B. A., Shannon, M. T., and Stang, C. L. (1994). *Govoni and Hayes: Nurses Drug Guide.* Norwalk, CT: Appleton and Lange.

Wyeth Laboratories (1988). *Intramuscular Injections.* Philadelphia: Wyeth Laboratories.

Zenk, K. E. (1980). Dosage calculations for drugs administered by infusion. *American Journal of Hospital Pharmacy.* 37:1304–1305.

Zenk, K. E. (1987). Intravenous drug delivery in infants with limited IV access and fluid restriction. *American Journal of Hospital Pharmacy.* 44(11):2542–2545.

Guidelines for Administration of Medications

ADMINISTRATION

ORAL MEDICATIONS

INJECTABLE MEDICATIONS

INTRAVENOUS FLOW AND MEDICATIONS

GENERAL DRUG ADMINISTRATION

1. Check medication order with doctor's orders, Kardex, medicine card (if available), and/or other methods.
2. Check label of drug container three times.
3. Check drug label for expiration date of *all* drugs. Return drugs that are outdated to the pharmacy.
4. Identify the patient by identification bracelet and by asking patient his or her name.
5. Stay with the patient until the medication is taken.
6. Give medications last to patients who need more assistance.
7. Report drug error immediately to the head nurse and physician. Incident report is necessary.
8. Record drug given, including the name of the drug, dosage, date, time, and your initials.
9. Record drugs soon after they are given, especially STAT medications. Also indicate on the drug sheet if the drug was not given.
10. Record oral intake of the amount of fluid taken with medication if the patient is on intake (I) and output (O).
11. Be aware that nurses have the right to question drug orders. Physicians are responsible for medication order, dosage, and route of drug administration. Nurses are responsible for administered medications.
12. Administer drug within 30 minutes of its prescribed time (30 minutes before or 30 minutes after prescribed time.
13. Do not guess when preparing medications. Check the order sheet if drug order is not clear. Call the pharmacist, physician, and/or nursing supervisor if in doubt.
14. Do not give drugs poured by others.
15. Do not leave drug tray or cart out of sight.
16. Know that patients have the right to refuse medication. If possible, ascertain why the patient refuses the medication. Report refusal to take medications.
17. Check if patient states that he or she has an allergy to a drug or a drug group.
18. Know the seven *rights:* right drug, right dose, right route, right time, right patient, right of patient to know reason for drug, and right of patient to refuse medication.

ORAL MEDICATIONS

1. Wash hands before preparing oral medications.
2. Pour tablet or capsule into drug container's cap (top) and *not* into the hand. Drugs prepared for unit dose can be opened at

the time of administration in the patient's room. Discard drugs that are dropped on the floor.

3. Pour liquids on a flat surface at eye level with your thumbnail on medicine cup line.

4. Do not mix liquids with tablets or liquids with liquids in the same container. Tablets and capsules can be put in the same container *except* for oral narcotics, digoxin, and PRN and STAT medications.

5. Do not pour drugs from containers with labels that are difficult to read.

6. Do not return poured medication to its container. Properly discard poured medication if not used.

7. Do not transfer medication from one container to another.

8. Pour liquid medications from the side opposite the bottle's label to avoid spilling medicine on the label.

9. Dilute liquid medications that irritate gastric mucosa, e.g., potassium products, or that could discolor or damage tooth enamel, e.g., SSKI, or have patient take the drug with meals.

10. Offer ice chips prior to distasteful medications to numb the patient's taste buds.

11. Assist the patient into upright position when administering oral medications. Stay with patient until medication is taken.

12. Give at least 50 to 100 mL of oral fluids with medications unless the patient has a fluid restriction. This helps to ensure that medication reaches the stomach.

13. For patients having difficulty in swallowing or for patients receiving nutrients through a nasogastric or gastric tube, crush tablets (*not* spansules) and dissolve in juice or applesauce for oral ingestion or water for tube administration. Give oral medication in small amounts to prevent choking. For the patient who has difficulty swallowing, gently stroke the throat in a downward motion to enhance swallowing.

14. For drugs given by oral syringe, direct the syringe across the tongue and toward the side of the mouth.

15. If a patient or a child spits out *all* of the liquid medication, repeat dose. When a patient or a child spits out more than one half of the liquid medication, repeat one half of the dose. If the patient or the child spits out less than one half of the liquid medication or if there is a question regarding redosing, the physician must be notified and another route of administration chosen.

INJECTABLE MEDICATIONS

1. Wash hands before preparing injectable medications.

2. Select the proper syringe and needle size for the type of medication to be administered.

3. Assess the degree of subcutaneous fat at the injection site before choosing the needle length for an intramuscular injection.

4. Select the injection site according to the drug.

5. Check for drug compatibility before mixing drugs in the same syringe.

6. Check the expiration date on the drug label before preparing medication. If in doubt, check with the pharmacist.

7. Check label on drug container to determine method(s) for drug administration, i.e., IM, IV, SC.

8. Do not give parenteral medications that are cloudy, are discolored, or have precipitated.

9. Aspirate plunger before injecting medication. If blood returns, *stop,* withdraw needle, and prepare new solution. Check the policy of your institution.

10. Do not massage injection site if using Z-track method, intradermal injection, heparin, or any anticoagulant solution.

11. Do not administer injections into inflamed and edematous tissues or into lesion (moles, birthmarks, scar) sites.

12. Recognize that individuals experiencing edema, shock, or poor circulation will have a very slow tissue absorption rate following intramuscular injection.

13. Discard liquid drugs into the sink or toilet, *not* into the trash can.

14. Discard needles safely into the proper container.

15. Refrigerate unused reconstituted powdered medication in vials. Write date, time, and initial on vial.

16. Discard unused solution in ampules. After they are opened, ampules cannot be reused.

17. Do not administer IM medications subcutaneously. Sloughing of the subcutaneous tissue could occur.

INTRAVENOUS FLOW AND MEDICATIONS

1. Wash hands before changing IV fluids and tubing and before preparing IV drugs.

2. Use aseptic technique when inserting IV catheter and changing IV tubing and bag. Recognize symptoms of septicemia, such as chills, fever, tachycardia.

3. Select appropriate IV tubing sets for continuous IV infusion. For IV fluids to infuse in 10 hours or *more,* use a microdrip set (60 gtt/min); for IV fluids to infuse in 10 hours or *less,* use a macrodrip set (10, 15, 20 gtt/min).

4. Add IV drugs such as vitamins and potassium chloride to the IV fluid before connecting the IV fluid to the IV tubing. Invert the IV

bag or bottle several times to ensure drug distribution. If the IV fluid is running and IV medication needs to be added, temporarily stop the IV fluid by clamping the tubing. Invert the IV bag or bottle several times, then unclamp the tubing and maintain the ordered IV flow rate.

5. Check for patency of IV catheter (heparin lock) before administering drugs by inserting 2 mL of saline solution. Flush IV line with 15 mL to empty the IV line of drug solution.

6. Use the proper diluent to reconstitute a powdered drug, and use the proper IV solution for infusion. Drug labels and drug circulars usually indicate the types of diluents to use.

7. Record on the vial containing unused drug the date of reconstitution and your initials.

8. Monitor all IV flow rates (conventional tubing or electronic IV regulators) hourly as needed. IV flow rates can alter owing to the patient's position or to a kink in the tubing.

9. Check for air bubbles in the IV tubing. Remove air from the tubing by clamping below the air bubbles and aspirating with a syringe or use the method that is indicated by your institution.

10. Assess for allergic reactions to the IV drug. If reactions are seen, stop flow rate of IV drug immediately.

11. Avoid administering drugs rapidly in IV solutions. Speed shock could occur as a result of drug concentration and accumulation. Symptoms can include tachycardia, syncope, and drop in blood pressure.

12. Observe the infusion site for signs of infiltration such as swelling, coolness, and pain. If these signs are observed, discontinue IV and restart at another site.

13. Assess for signs and symptoms of phlebitis such as redness, warmth, swelling, and pain. Redness may be seen above the infusion site along the vein.

14. Do not forcefully irrigate IV catheters. Clots can be dislodged from the catheter site and become an embolus.

15. Avoid leg veins, elbow (antecubital) site, and affected limbs for use in IV therapy.

16. Change IV site every 3 days or as indicated. Certain IV catheters, such as polyethylene catheters, can cause phlebitis.

17. Change IV tubing every 24–48 hours, and change IV bag every 24 hours.

18. Apply cold compresses followed later by warm compresses to hematoma site, according to the physician's orders.

Nomograms

BODY SURFACE AREA
FOR ADULTS NOMOGRAM

WEST NOMOGRAM FOR
INFANTS AND CHILDREN

BODY SURFACE AREA FOR ADULTS – NOMOGRAM

HEIGHT	BODY SURFACE AREA (BSA)	WEIGHT

HEIGHT	BSA	WEIGHT
cm 200 — 79 inch	2.80 m²	kg 150 — 330 lb
78	2.70	145 — 320
195 — 77	2.60	140 — 310
76		135 — 300
190 — 75	2.50	130 — 290
74		125 — 280
185 — 73	2.40	270
72		120 — 260
180 — 71	2.30	115 — 250
70		110 — 240
175 — 69	2.20	105 — 230
68		100 — 220
170 — 67	2.10	
66		95 — 210
165 — 65	2.00	90 — 200
64	1.95	
160 — 63	1.90	85 — 190
62	1.85	80 — 180
155 — 61	1.80	170
60	1.75	75 — 160
150 — 59	1.70	70 — 150
58	1.65	
145 — 57	1.60	65 — 140
56	1.55	60 — 130
140 — 55	1.50	
54	1.45	55 — 120
135 — 53	1.40	50 — 110
52	1.35	105
130 — 51	1.30	45 — 100
50		95
125 — 49	1.25	40 — 90
48	1.20	85
120 — 47	1.15	35 — 80
46	1.10	75
115 — 45	1.05	70
44	1.00	kg 30 — 66 lb
110 — 43	0.95	
42	0.90	
105 — 41	0.86 m²	
40		
cm 100 — 39 in		

Body Surface Area (BSA) Nomogram for Adults

Directions: (1) Find height. (2) Find weight. (3) Draw a straight line connecting the height and weight. Where the line intersects on the BSA column is the body surface area (m²). (From Deglin, J. H., Vallerand, A. H., and Russin, M. M. (1991). *Davis's Drug Guide for Nurses,* 2nd ed. Philadelphia: F. A. Davis, p. 1218. Used with permission from Lentner C. (ed.) (1981). *Geigy Scientific Tables,* 8th ed., Vol. 1. Basel, Switzerland: Ciba-Geigy, pp. 226–227.

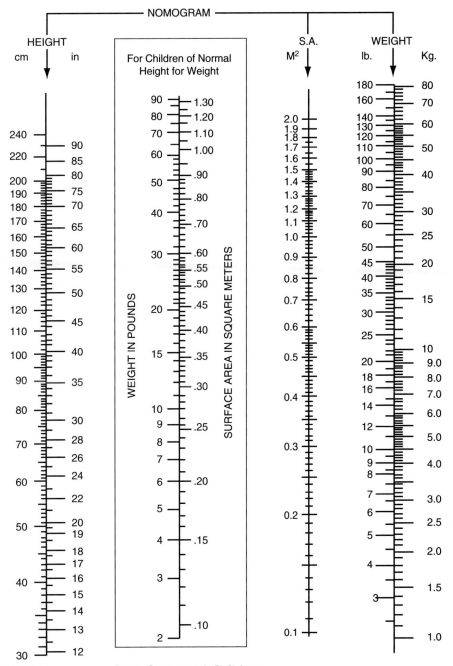

West Nomogram for Infants and Children

Directions: (1) Find height. (2) Find weight. (3) Draw a straight line connecting the height and weight. Where the line intersects on the SA column is the body surface area (m²). (Modified from data of E. Boyd and C. D. West, in Behrman, R. E. and Vaughan, V. C. (1992). *Nelson Textbook of Pediatrics*, 14th ed. Philadelphia, W. B. Saunders.)

INDEX

Abbreviations

cc	= mL (milliliter)
mL	= cc (cubic centimeter)
fl dr	= fl ʒ
fl oz	= fl ℥
g, Gm	= gram
gr	= grain
gtt	= drops
kg	= kilogram
mcg, μg	= microgram
mg	= milligram
l, L	= liter
ss	= one-half
T	= tablespoon
t	= teaspoon
A.D.	= right ear
O.D.	= right eye
A.S.	= left ear
O.S.	= left eye
A.U.	= both ears
O.U.	= both eyes
<	= less than
>	= greater than

Drug Calculations
Basic Formula

$$\frac{D \text{ (desired)}}{H \text{ (on hand)}} \times V \text{ (vehicle, drug form)}$$

Example:

Order: amoxicillin 100 mg, po, q6h.
Available: amoxicillin 250 mg/5 mL

$$\frac{D}{H} \times V = \frac{100 \text{ mg}}{250 \text{ mg}} \times 5 \text{ mL}$$

$$= \frac{500}{250} = 2 \text{ mL amoxicillin}$$

METRIC AND APOTHECARY CONVERSION

Metric		Apothecary
Gram (g)	Milligram (mg)	Grain (gr)
1	1000	15
0.5	500	7½
0.3	300 (325)	5
0.1	100	1½
0.06	60 (64)	1
0.03	30 (32)	½
0.015	15 (16)	¼
0.010	10	⅙
0.0006	0.6	1/100
0.0004	0.4	1/150
0.0003	0.3	1/200

Volume/Hour (mL/hr)

$$\frac{\text{concentration/hr}}{\text{concentration of solution}} = \text{mL/hr}$$

$$\frac{\text{(mg, mcg, U)/hr}}{\text{(mg, mcg, U)/mL}} = \text{mL/hr}$$

or

If volume/min is known, multiply volume/min by 60 minutes = mL/hr

Drug Calculations
Ratio and Proportion:

$$H \quad : \quad V \quad :: \quad D \quad \quad X$$
on hand vehicle desired unknown

means

extremes

Example:

Order: amoxicillin 100 mg, po, q6h
Available: amoxicillin 250 mg/5 mL

$$H \quad : \quad V \quad :: \quad D \quad : \quad X$$
$$250 \text{ mg} : 5 \text{ mL} :: 100 \text{ mg} : X \text{ mL}$$

$$250 \text{ X} = 500$$
$$X = 2 \text{ mL amoxicillin}$$

IV Flow Rate: Continuous
Method III:

$$\frac{\text{amount of fluid} \times \text{gtt/mL (IV set)}}{\text{hours to administer} \times \text{min/hr (60)}} = \text{gtt/min}$$

Example:

Order: 1000 mL of D_5W over 10 hours.
IV Set: microdrip 60 gtt/mL.

$$\frac{\overset{100}{\cancel{1000}} \text{ mL} \times \overset{1}{\cancel{60}} \text{ gtt/mL}}{\underset{1}{\cancel{10}} \text{ hours} \times \underset{1}{\cancel{60}} \text{ min/hr}} = 100 \text{ gtt/min}$$

Concentration/Hour in
(mg, mcg, U)/hr

concentration/min $\times$ 60 min/hr
(mg, mcg, U)/min $\times$ 60 min/hr

or

concentration of solution $\times$ volume/hr
(mg, mcg, U)/mL $\times$ mL/hr

Basic Fractional Formula

$$\frac{\text{concentration of solution}}{\text{drop rate of set}} = \frac{\text{desired concentration/min} \times \text{wt in kg}}{\text{volume/hr or gtt/min}}$$

$$\frac{\text{(mg, mcg, U)/mL}}{60 \text{ gtt/mL*}} = \frac{\text{(mg, mcg, U)/min}}{\text{mL/hr}}$$

* 60 gtt/mL is constant.
  Two other quantities must be known.
  The unknown quantity can be X.

Right Time

· Administer drug at the specified time(s). ☐
· Document any delay or omitted drug dose. ☐
· Administer drugs that irritate gastric mucosa ☐
  with food.
· Administer antibiotics at even intervals (q6h, ☐
  q8h).

Right Route

· Know the route for administration of the ☐
  drug.
· Use aseptic techniques when administering a ☐
  drug.
· Document the injection site on the patient's ☐
  chart.

$$\textbf{Volume/min} = \textbf{mL/min}$$

$$\frac{\text{Concentration/min}}{\text{Concentration of solution}}$$

$$\frac{\text{mg, mcg, units/min}}{\text{mg/mL}}$$

or

$$\frac{\text{Volume/hr}}{60 \text{ min}}$$

If volume/hr is known set up a ratio and proportion:

Volume : 60 min = X mL : mL

Concentration/Minute in (mg, mcg, U)/min

Concentration of solution $\times$ volume/min
(mg, mcg, U)/mL $\times$ mL/min

or

$$\frac{\text{concentration/hr}}{60 \text{ min/hr}}$$

$$\frac{(\text{mg, mcg, U})/\text{hr}}{60 \text{ min/hr}}$$

Checklist of the "Five Rights" in Drug Administration

Right Client
- Check client's identification bracelet. ☐
- Ask the client for his or her name. ☐
- Check name on the client's medication label. ☐

Right Drug
- Check that the drug order is complete and legible. ☐
- Check the drug label 3 times. ☐
- Check the expiration date. ☐
- Know the drug action. ☐

Right Dose
- Calculate the drug dose. ☐
- Know the recommended dosage range for the drug. ☐
- Recalculate drug dose with another nurse if in doubt. ☐